Guideline Development and Implementation in Rheumatic Disease

Editor

MICHAEL M. WARD

RHEUMATIC DISEASE CLINICS OF NORTH AMERICA

www.rheumatic.theclinics.com

Consulting Editor
MICHAEL H. WEISMAN

August 2022 • Volume 48 • Number 3

ELSEVIER

1600 John F. Kennedy Boulevard ● Suite 1800 ● Philadelphia, Pennsylvania, 19103-2899
http://www.theclinics.com

RHEUMATIC DISEASE CLINICS OF NORTH AMERICA Volume 48, Number 3
August 2022 ISSN 0889-857X, ISBN 13: 978-0-323-96048-9

Editor: Joanna Collett
Developmental Editor: Karen Solomon

Rheumatic Disease Clinics of North America (ISSN 0889-857X) is published quarterly by Elsevier Inc., 360 Park Avenue South, New York, NY 10010-1710. Months of issue are February, May, August, and November. Business and editorial offices: 1600 John F. Kennedy Boulevard, Suite 1800, Philadelphia, PA 19103-2899. Periodicals postage paid at New York, NY and additional mailing offices. Subscription prices are USD 366.00 per year for US individuals, USD 1020.00 per year for US institutions, USD 100.00 per year for US students and residents, USD 431.00 per year for Canadian individuals, USD 1040.00 per year for Canadian institutions, USD 100.00 per year for Canadian students/residents, USD 470.00 per year for international individuals, USD 1040.00 per year for international institutions, and USD 230.00 per year for foreign students/residents. To receive student/ resident rate, orders must be accompanied by name of affiliated institution, date of term, and the *signature* of program/residency coordinator on institution letterhead. Orders will be billed at individual rate until proof of status received. Foreign air speed delivery is included in all *Clinics* subscription prices. All prices are subject to change without notice. **POSTMASTER:** Send address changes to *Rheumatic Disease Clinics of North America,* Elsevier Health Sciences Division, Subscription Customer Service, 3251 Riverport Lane, Maryland Heights, MO 63043. **Customer Service: 1-800-654-2452 (US and Canada). From outside of the US and Canada: 314-447-8871. Fax: 314-447-8029. For print support, e-mail: JournalsCustomerService-usa@elsevier.com. For online support, e-mail: JournalsOnlineSupport-usa@elsevier.com.**

Reprints. For copies of 100 or more of articles in this publication, please contact the Commercial Reprints Department, Elsevier Inc., 360 Park Avenue South, New York, New York, 10010-1710; Tel.: +1-212-633-3874, Fax: +1-212-633-3820, and E-mail: reprints@elsevier.com.

Rheumatic Disease Clinics of North America is covered in *MEDLINE/PubMed (Index Medicus), Current Contents/Clinical Medicine, Science Citation Index, ISI/BIOMED,* and *EMBASE/Excerpta Medica.*

Contributors

CONSULTING EDITOR

MICHAEL H. WEISMAN, MD
Adjunct Professor of Medicine, Stanford University, Distinguished Professor of Medicine, Emeritus, David Geffen School of Medicine at UCLA, Professor of Medicine Emeritus, Cedars-Sinai Medical Center, Los Angeles, California, USA

EDITOR

MICHAEL M. WARD, MD, MPH
National Institute of Arthritis and Musculoskeletal and Skin Diseases, Bethesda, Maryland, USA

AUTHORS

CLAIRE E.H. BARBER, MD, PhD, FRCPC
Associate Professor, Departments of Medicine and Community Health Sciences, Cumming School of Medicine, University of Calgary, Calgary, Alberta, Canada; Research Scientist, Arthritis Research Canada, Vancouver, British Columbia, Canada

CHERYL BARNABE, MD, MSc, FRCPC
Professor, Departments of Medicine and Community Health Sciences, Cumming School of Medicine, University of Calgary, Calgary, Alberta, Canada; Research Scientist, Arthritis Research Canada, Vancouver, British Columbia, Canada

GEORGE BERTSIAS, MD, PhD
Rheumatology and Clinical Immunology, University of Crete Medical School, Institute of Molecular Biology and Biotechnology, Foundation for Research and Technology – Hellas (FORTH), Heraklion, Greece

HERMINE I. BRUNNER, MD, MBA
Professor of Pediatrics, Cincinnati Children's Medical Center and University of Cincinnati, Cincinnati, Ohio, USA

AYDIA MAYAN CAPLAN
Research Student, Rocky Mountain Regional Veterans Affairs Medical Center, University of Colorado Anschutz Medical Campus, Aurora, Colorado, USA

LIRON CAPLAN, MD, PhD
Rheumatology Section Head, Rocky Mountain Regional Veterans Affairs Medical Center, University of Colorado Anschutz Medical Campus, Aurora, Colorado, USA

KIRAN DHIMAN, MPH
Research Coordinator, Department of Medicine, Cumming School of Medicine, University of Calgary, Calgary, Alberta, Canada

ANISHA B. DUA, MD, MPH
Associate Professor of Medicine, Northwestern University Feinberg School of Medicine, Chicago, Illinois, USA

ALLAN C. GELBER, MD, MPH, PhD
Professor of Medicine, Division of Rheumatology, Department of Medicine, Johns Hopkins School of Medicine, Department of Epidemiology, Johns Hopkins Bloomberg School of Public Health, Baltimore, Maryland, USA

SUSAN M. GOODMAN, MD
Professor of Clinical Medicine, Hospital for Special Surgery, Weill Cornell Medicine, New York, New York, USA

NICOLE M.S. HARTFELD, MSc, MC, CCC
Research Coordinator, Department of Medicine, Cumming School of Medicine, University of Calgary, Calgary, Alberta, Canada

GLEN S. HAZLEWOOD, MD, PhD, FRCPC
Associate Professor, Departments of Medicine and Community Health Sciences, Cumming School of Medicine, University of Calgary, Calgary, Alberta, Canada; Research Scientist, Arthritis Research Canada, Vancouver, British Columbia, Canada

SINDHU R. JOHNSON, MD, PhD
Associate Professor of Medicine, Division of Rheumatology, Department of Medicine, Toronto Western Hospital, Mount Sinai Hospital, Institute of Health Policy, Management and Evaluation, University of Toronto, Toronto, Ontario, Canada

TANAZ A. KERMANI, MD, MS
Associate Clinical Professor of Medicine, University of California, Los Angeles, Santa Monica, California, USA

UNA E. MAKRIS, MD, MSc
Associate Professor, UT Southwestern Medical Center, VA North Texas Health System, Dallas, Texas, USA

JAMAL MIKDASHI, MD, MPH
Associate Professor of Medicine, Division of Rheumatology and Clinical Immunology, University of Maryland School of Medicine, Baltimore, Maryland, USA

AMANDA E. NELSON, MD, MSCR
Division of Rheumatology, Allergy, and Immunology, Thurston Arthritis Research Center, The University of North Carolina at Chapel Hill, Chapel Hill, North California, USA

TUHINA NEOGI, MD, PhD
Boston University School of Medicine, Boston, Massachusetts, USA

EKEMINI A. OGBU, MD, MSc
Assistant Professor of Pediatrics, Cincinnati Children's Medical Center and University of Cincinnati, Cincinnati, Ohio, USA; Adjunct Assistant Professor of Pediatrics, Johns Hopkins University, Baltimore, Maryland, USA

CHRIS OVERTON, MD
Division of Rheumatology, Allergy, and Immunology, Thurston Arthritis Research Center, The University of North Carolina at Chapel Hill, Chapel Hill, North California, USA

JASVINDER A. SINGH, MBBS, MPH
Medicine Service, VA Medical Center, Professor of Medicine and Epidemiology,
Department of Medicine at the School of Medicine, University of Alabama at Birmingham,
Department of Epidemiology, University of Alabama at Birmingham School of Public
Health, Birmingham, Alabama, USA

LISA G. SUTER, MD
Professor of Medicine (Rheumatology), Yale School of Medicine, New Haven,
Connecticut, USA; Connecticut Veterans Health Administration, West Haven,
Connecticut, USA

AMY S. TURNER
Senior Director, Quality, American College of Rheumatology, Atlanta, Georgia, USA

ELIZABETH WAHL, MD, MAS
Department of Medicine, Division of Rheumatology, Acting Division Chief and Assistant
Professor, University of Washington, VA Puget Sound Healthcare System, Seattle,
Washington, USA

KENNETH J. WARRINGTON, MD
Professor of Medicine, Mayo Clinic, Rochester, Minnesota, USA

Contents

Clinical practice guidelines are important documents developed and endorsed by the American College of Rheumatology to support its membership and other clinicians in the care of patients with rheumatic and musculoskeletal diseases. Clinical practice guidelines serve several roles including guiding health care professionals on treatment of a disease, screening, and/or diagnosis. Rigorously developed guidelines are based on the most recent scientific evidence, in consultation with experts, including patients. This article discusses the purpose of clinical practice guidelines, highlighting their strengths and limitations. Policies and procedures of the American College of Rheumatology for the development and endorsement of guidelines are summarized.

The Grades of Recommendation, Assessment, Development and Evaluation (GRADE) approach has emerged as an extremely common method for rating quality of a body of evidence in systematic reviews and for converting this evidence into guidelines. The American College of Rheumatology has effectively adopted this method, with minor modifications, for recent guidelines. This article reviews some of the basic principles of the GRADE approach and provides additional resources for use of GRADE.

Quality measures (QMs) are tools that help measure or quantify health care processes, outcomes, patient perceptions, and organizational structures and systems associated with the ability to provide high-quality health care. QMs are often developed from clinical practice guidelines (CPGs), as they summarize the best available evidence to create standards for optimizing patient care. The authors provide a framework for learners to understand the relevance, development, and testing of QMs in rheumatology, touching on their relationship to CPGs and appropriate use criteria. They describe measure implementation across different health care settings and reflect on challenges and opportunities associated with this process.

Since the first systemic lupus erythematosus (SLE) guidelines published by the American College of Rheumatology in 1999, accumulating data from observational and randomized-controlled studies, including the advent of biological agents, have stimulated the production of recommendations by various committees and task forces. Still, several areas relating to the diagnosis, treatment, and monitoring of SLE remain uncertain due to limited or inconclusive evidence, therefore emphasizing the role of expert consensus in reaching balanced and informative statements. This review outlines the most recent SLE recommendations highlighting key differences and important challenges that will also need to be considered in future updates.

Despite the high prevalence and burden of osteoarthritis (OA) worldwide, management of OA continues to primarily focus on symptom management due to the lack of approved pharmacologic agents that halt disease progression. Recent recommendations from 6 professional societies support the importance of education, self-management approaches, weight loss, and physical modalities in managing OA. These recent guidelines also highlight the paucity of effective and safe treatment options, with recommendations against ineffective therapies outnumbering those for effective ones. NSAIDs, oral and topical, remain the primary recommended pharmacologic management option for OA.

The range of drug treatment options to treat acute and chronic gout has changed dramatically over the last 20 years. Yet, there is general consensus that drug therapy selection, dosing and dose titration, of both traditional and novel agents is far from optimally delivered in clinical practice. Updated guidelines disseminated in the last 5 years, from the American College of Physicians, the European League Against Rheumatism, and the American College of Rheumatology, provide clear guidance to the medical community on how and when to optimally integrate these therapeutic options into practice to improve the medical management of gout.

Rheumatoid arthritis is the most common autoimmune, destructive, inflammatory arthritis in adults. Effective treatments include oral conventional synthetic disease-modifying antirheumatic drugs (DMARDs; eg, methotrexate), injectable biologic DMARDs, and targeted synthetic DMARDs (oral). Key recommendations are to start effective treatment immediately with DMARDs to reduce disability; use effective doses of methotrexate (oral or subcutaneous) with folic acid as the initial treatment; rapidly escalate treatment with various DMARDs, if methotrexate alone is not effective in controlling rheumatoid arthritis; and aim for a treat-to-target strategy with a goal of low disease activity or remission by frequently monitoring disease activity and escalating treatment.

Patient participation is an integral component in the development of clinical practice guidelines. However, patient engagement remains suboptimal, which signifies a predicament in guideline's legitimacy and transparency. Limited budgets, logistic constraints, and discordance in patients' and researchers' perception of a meaningful involvement are some barriers that hinder patient engagement. Advancing skill development across various roles within the guideline's process will enrich patient's contribution and allow them to voice their experience, knowledge, perspective, and concerns. Continuing patient education and evaluation of their engagement on both outcome and process will facilitate team cohesion, trustworthiness, and value to achieve optimal quality of care.

The vasculitides encompass a group of inflammatory conditions affecting the blood vessels with severe consequences including tissue ischemia, structural abnormalities, such as aneurysms/dissections, and end organ damage. The different forms are commonly classified based on the size of the blood vessel involved as large-vessel, medium-vessel, and small-vessel vasculitis. The American College of Rheumatology/Vasculitis Foundation recently published guidelines on the management of several forms of primary systemic vasculitides. In this review, the recommendations for giant cell arteritis, Takayasu arteritis, polyarteritis nodosa, granulomatosis with polyangiitis, microscopic polyangiitis, and eosinophilic granulomatosis with polyangiitis are discussed. We highlight the key recommendations, aspects where they diverge from other published guidelines, controversies, and areas of uncertainty.

Treatment guidelines provide strategies for managing specific disease conditions based on the best scientific evidence available. Pediatric rheumatologists manage predominantly rare autoimmune and autoinflammatory conditions. Although the availability of guidelines to inform treatment decisions in pediatric rheumatic diseases is desirable, only a few treatment guidelines exist. Furthermore, the rarity of these diseases limits the feasibility of conducting randomized controlled studies to inform guideline recommendations. Thus, there remains a need for stronger supporting evidence for recommendations, and treatment guidelines for rarer rheumatologic diseases. In this review, we give an overview of past and current guidelines in pediatric rheumatology.

We evaluated the quality of selected rheumatology guidelines using the Appraisal of Guidelines for Research and Evaluation (AGREE) II instrument. Guidelines were also assessed to determine if Grading of Recommendations Assessment, Development, and Evaluation (GRADE) methodology had been used during development and for the inclusion of health inequity considerations. Only half of the guidelines used the GRADE methodology, and this was associated with higher AGREE II ratings in the Rigor of Development domain. Ongoing areas identified for improvement included more meaningful engagement of patients in guideline panels, increased transparency of the management of conflicts of interest, improved reporting of strategies for guideline implementation, and increased consideration of the health equity implications throughout guideline development and implementation.

RHEUMATIC DISEASE CLINICS OF NORTH AMERICA

SERIES OF RELATED INTEREST

Medical Clinics of North America
https://www.medical.theclinics.com/
Neurologic Clinics
https://www.neurologic.theclinics.com/
Dermatologic Clinics
https://www.derm.theclinics.com/
Physical Medicine and Rehabilitation Clinics of North America
https://www.pmr.theclinics.com/

THE CLINICS ARE AVAILABLE ONLINE!
Access your subscription at:
www.theclinics.com

Foreword

Guideline Development and Implementation in Rheumatic Disease

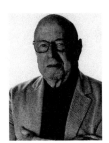

Michael H. Weisman, MD
Consulting Editor

Dr Ward has assembled a series of outstanding articles describing clinical practice guidelines (CPG) and treatment recommendations that have evolved over the past decade. Methodologies have been standardized for the approaches that create the GCPs, and there have been attempts, mostly successful, to eliminate bias and provide transparency so that the reader can determine how to best incorporate them into their professional lives. He has also provided the reader with articles that describe the methods by which these guidelines can be fit into institutional practices and policy decisions to develop uniformity in their application that will improve quality of care. Words of caution were also expressed by our contributors related to ongoing areas identified for improvement. These included but were not limited to more meaningful engagement of patients in guideline panels, increased transparency of the management of conflicts of interest, improved reporting of strategies for guideline implementation, and increased consideration of the health equity implications throughout guideline development and implementation.

There is a need to address how the CPG and treatment recommendations fare in the educational process of our Fellows in Rheumatology; this is an area that needs discussion and more work. We teach that the highest level of allegiance to guidelines relate to their fidelity as representing data from well-controlled clinical trials in patients who fit strict classification criteria. However, should we rely on that guideline to decide how to treat that sick patient in the hospital with ambiguous overlapping clinical and laboratory aspects of different rheumatic diseases (features that would have excluded that

Rheum Dis Clin N Am 48 (2022) xiii–xiv
https://doi.org/10.1016/j.rdc.2022.06.013
0889-857X/22/© 2022 Published by Elsevier Inc.

rheumatic.theclinics.com

patient from the trials in the first place)? More work needs to be done to recognize the strengths and limitations of what we have created.

Michael H. Weisman, MD
10800 Wilshire Boulevard, #404
Los Angeles, CA 90024, USA

E-mail address:
michael.weisman@cshs.org

Preface

A Guide to Contemporary Clinical Practice Guidelines

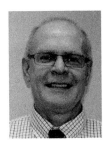

Michael M. Ward, MD, MPH
Editor

Over the past 15 years, clinical practice guidelines (CPG), or treatment recommendations, have come to occupy a prominent place in the care of patients, the education of trainees, and the work of professional societies. CPGs were borne out of the movement to evidence-based medicine and the resultant need to identify, organize, summarize, and evaluate the exploding medical literature for busy clinicians who may not have the time or methodological training to do so independently. Because evidence-based medicine places controlled trials at the top of the evidence hierarchy, clinical questions that have been addressed by one or more clinical trials tend to have CPGs of high confidence. Unfortunately, and particularly for less prevalent rheumatic diseases, many important clinical questions have not been addressed by clinical trials. In these instances, CPGs try to integrate the best available observational evidence with the opinions and experience of disease experts, including patients. The ideal of CPGs is to provide trustworthy, expert, current, and unbiased treatment recommendations for commonly encountered clinical scenarios.

This issue includes articles on 2 themes: the process and methods of generating GCPs, and reviews of current CPGs in several rheumatic diseases. The issue starts with an overview of the processes used by the American College of Rheumatology (ACR) in developing their CPGs, followed by a discussion of how CPGs relate to, and differ from, 2 other practice metrics, quality indicators and appropriateness criteria. Next, the Grading of Recommendations, Assessment, Development, and Evaluation method, which is the current standard for rating the quality of evidence in the literature and translating this into recommendations, is explained. The involvement of patients in the formulation of CPGs has increasingly been recognized as essential for relevance and quality, and the challenges and opportunities for greater patient participation are discussed in the following article.

Rheum Dis Clin N Am 48 (2022) xv–xvi
https://doi.org/10.1016/j.rdc.2022.06.012
0889-857X/22/© 2022 Published by Elsevier Inc.

rheumatic.theclinics.com

The disease-specific articles provide critical appraisals of current CPGs in many of the major rheumatic diseases: osteoarthritis of the knee, hip, and hands; rheumatoid arthritis; gout; systemic lupus erythematosus; systemic vasculitis; and pediatric rheumatic diseases. When available, authors have contrasted recommendations from different professional societies, demonstrating instances where differences may result from considerations applied to the same body of literature. It is important to note that although some of the content in this issue relates to ACR products and some authors have participated in ACR product development, the articles in this issue reflect the experience, expertise, and opinions of the authors and are not official ACR products.

The concluding article details the approaches used to evaluate the quality of CPGs, reminding us that the raters also get rated. The goal of this quality check is again to assess the trustworthiness of CGPs, and if necessary, stimulate improvement in the future. We hope that this issue helps familiarize readers with both the process and the content of CPGs so readers can determine how to best incorporate them in their practice.

Michael M. Ward, MD, MPH
National Institute of Arthritis and
Musculoskeletal and Skin Diseases
Building 10CRC, Room 4-1339
10 Center Drive
Bethesda, MD 20892, USA

E-mail address:
Wardm1@mail.nih.gov

How the American College of Rheumatology Develops Guidelines

Sindhu R. Johnson, MD, PhD[a],*, Amy S. Turner[b],
Susan M. Goodman, MD[c]

KEYWORDS

- Guidelines • Clinical practice • Evidence

KEY POINTS

- Clinical practice guidelines are intended to promote desirable outcomes but cannot guarantee any specific outcome.
- The American College of Rheumatology places a high priority on developing methodologically rigorous, evidence-based clinical practice guidelines that take into consideration the expertise and viewpoints of multiple stakeholders in a transparent fashion.
- Recommendations are characterized by strength (as either strong or conditional) and the quality of evidence supporting them (rated as high, moderate, low, or very low).

INTRODUCTION
What Is the Purpose of Clinical Practice Guidelines?

Clinical practice guidelines are among the most important documents developed and endorsed by the American College of Rheumatology (ACR) to support its membership and other clinicians in the care of patients with rheumatic and musculoskeletal diseases. Clinical practice guidelines serve several roles[1] including guiding health care professionals on treatment of a disease (and sometimes also screening and/or diagnosis) and, therefore, making them better health care providers. Rigorously developed guidelines are based on the most recent scientific evidence, in consultation with experts, including patients. Guidelines may serve several other purposes:

- Guidelines may result in a reduction in geographic practice variation and inappropriate care.
- Guidelines are used for advocacy, to promote disease awareness or advocate for improved access to medical testing (eg, imaging) or treatments.

[a] Division of Rheumatology, Department of Medicine, Toronto Western Hospital, Mount Sinai Hospital, Institute of Health Policy, Management and Evaluation, University of Toronto, Room 2-004, Box 9, 60 Murray Street, Toronto, Ontario M5T 3L9, Canada; [b] American College of Rheumatology, 2200 Lake Blvd NE, Atlanta, GA 30319, USA; [c] Hospital for Special Surgery, 535 East 70th Street, 5th Floor, New York, NY 10021, USA
* Corresponding author.
E-mail address: Sindhu.Johnson@uhn.ca

Rheum Dis Clin N Am 48 (2022) 579–588
https://doi.org/10.1016/j.rdc.2022.04.001
0889-857X/22/© 2022 Elsevier Inc. All rights reserved.

- Guidelines may facilitate better access to government resources and/or influence partner organizations.
- Guidelines can help set clear policy for the organization that developed the guideline or other organizations that might use the guideline by providing an objective foundation for policy decisions.
- Guidelines may inform organizational communications with patients or allocation of resources.

Words of Caution

When considering a guideline, readers should be aware of a few cautionary notes. These documents are usually region specific. In the case of the ACR guidelines, they are intended for use in the United States and are developed in the context of Food and Drug Administration utilization approvals or restrictions. Guidelines have also been criticized for how race is considered.[2] There are no race reporting standards, and guidelines frequently rely on studies in populations with little racial or ethnic diversity. More recently, ACR guidelines have made race-based recommendations for areas where evidence is available (eg, testing for HLA-B*5801 allele before starting allopurinol is conditionally recommended for patients of South Asian descent [eg, Han Chinese, Korean, Thai] and African American patients, over not testing for the HLA-B*5801 allele).[3]

ACR disclaimer language on its guidelines includes that "guidelines and recommendations developed and/or endorsed by the ACR are intended to provide guidance for particular patterns of practice" and common medical scenarios, "not to dictate the care of a particular patient" or be used in all clinical situations.[1] These documents are not intended to be used to withhold care from a patient.

Guidelines require considerable resources to develop. These are frequently multi-year projects, requiring highly skilled professional and face-to-face (in-person or virtual) meetings. Guidelines are threatened by becoming outdated soon after or sometimes even before they are published.[4] Maintenance of the guidelines requires that the developers be nimble. Ideally, guidelines should be modified in a timely manner without loss of rigor. This too requires the time of highly skilled personnel. Finally, as the ACR notes, "guidelines are intended to promote desirable outcomes but cannot guarantee any specific outcome."[1] The ACR uses the Grading of Recommendations Assessment, Development, and Evaluation (GRADE) system for transparency in rating the quality of the evidence and the strength of the recommendations,[5] but recommendations cannot adequately convey all uncertainties and nuances of decisions regarding patient care (**Boxes 1** and **2**).

AMERICAN COLLEGE OF RHEUMATOLOGY POLICIES AND PROCEDURES

The ACR has a standardized process for the development and endorsement of clinical practice guidelines (**Fig. 1**). In this article we provide a summary of this process.

Box 1
Clinical practice guidelines: benefits

Benefits/intentions
- Provide guidance to health care professionals on treatment (and/or screening)
- Used to advocate for disease awareness and improved access to care
- Facilitate better access to government resources and/or influence partner organizations
- Help set clear policy
- Promote desirable outcomes

> **Box 2**
> **Clinical practice guidelines: challenges**
>
> Challenges/limitations
> - Are not designed to provide recommendations for patients in all geographic regions
> - Should not be used to withhold care from a patient
> - Require considerable resources to develop and maintain (eg, experts, financial support, time)
> - Cannot guarantee any specific outcome

Additional details are found in the ACR Guideline Manual, which is freely available on the ACR Web site.[1]

Define the Area

The first step is to define the area for which there is a need for guideline, such as the treatment of gout,[3] the treatment of rheumatoid arthritis,[6] or perioperative management of antirheumatic medication in patients with rheumatic and musculoskeletal diseases undergoing total hip or knee arthroplasty.[7] The ACR Guideline Subcommittee recommends topics to the ACR Committee on Quality of Care (QOC), based partly on needs expressed by the ACR membership, the broader rheumatology community, and/or ACR leadership. All topic suggestions are considered at the fall Guideline Subcommittee meeting, and decisions are made about which topics to recommend to QOC for inclusion in the next year's budget. In January, the QOC considers the Guideline Subcommittee's proposed topics as part of its budgetary process and decides about recommending proposed topics to the ACR Board of Directors for funding approval. If the QOC desires possible involvement of another organization in either the guideline development or approval process, the QOC requests Board approval of that relationship at the time of project approval so the relationship can be initiated, and its parameters established before the project begins.

After ACR Board of Directors approval of the topic and related project budget, the Guideline Subcommittee develops a Call for Letters of Interest (LOI). The LOI and project timeline are posted on the ACR Web site and distributed electronically to the ACR membership. The Call for LOI includes the guideline purpose, scope, audience, and estimated timeline; an explanation of the research methods to be used for guideline development; and a list of affected companies.

The guideline project development group is formed from the pool of LOIs, and additional suggestions made by Guideline Subcommittee or QOC members. (**Table 1**) The ACR goal is to include all stakeholders in as diverse a team as possible, such as:

- Rheumatologists, other physicians, specialists, and health professionals who care for patients with the target disease
- Private practitioners and academicians
- At least one clinician or clinical epidemiologist with significant GRADE methodology expertise and experience
- Patients with the diseases that are the topic of the guideline (and parents/caregivers, if the guideline topic is pediatric)

Several additional factors are taken into consideration. Individuals with the necessary clinical expertise, methodologic expertise, range or stage of career, sex, and geographic representation and potential conflicts of interest are all considered. The expertise of other relevant stakeholders is also incorporated.

A core leadership team of four to six people is confirmed to lead the work of the project with ACR staff. The project principal investigator (PI) may also serve as the

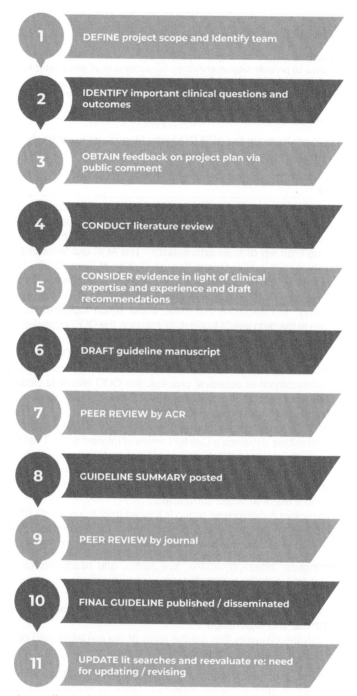

1   DEFINE project scope and Identify team

2   IDENTIFY important clinical questions and outcomes

3   OBTAIN feedback on project plan via public comment

4   CONDUCT literature review

5   CONSIDER evidence in light of clinical expertise and experience and draft recommendations

6   DRAFT guideline manuscript

7   PEER REVIEW by ACR

8   GUIDELINE SUMMARY posted

9   PEER REVIEW by journal

10   FINAL GUIDELINE published / disseminated

11   UPDATE lit searches and reevaluate re: need for updating / revising

Fig. 1. American College of Rheumatology clinical practice guideline development process.

Table 1
The guideline development group

Term	Definition
Guideline development group	Includes anyone intellectually involved in the development of ACR guidelines. Includes but may not be limited to core leadership team members, literature review team members, and voting panel members.
Principal investigator	The individual (usually a clinician) who leads an ACR guideline development project.
Core leadership team	4–6 individuals with content and methodologic expertise who oversee the project with ACR staff. At minimum, includes: 1. Project PI, who is primarily accountable with ACR staff for the completion of the work according to the agreed on project plan and timeline. 2. Literature review leader, who with the literature review team is responsible for conducting a systematic literature review and developing an evidence report. The literature review team leader may come from within the ACR or from an outside organization. 3. A guideline panel leader, who leads the decision process regarding the recommendations (may be the project PI, or a different person). 4. A GRADE expert.
Literature review team	The group of people who conduct the systematic review of available evidence that serves as the basis of the recommendations made in the guideline.
Patient panel	10–12 patients (including parents/caregivers, if a pediatric guideline) who discuss patient values and preferences related to outcomes, evidence, and drafted recommendation statements. Two patient panelists also sit on the voting panel to represent the views of the patient panel in voting discussions and decisions, which take into consideration trade-offs between the benefits and harms of alternative management strategies.
Voting panel	10–12 individuals who are responsible for analyzing available evidence and considering patient values and preferences in the context of their own experience and expertise, and then voting on the final recommendations.
Expert panel (optional)	Individuals with particular expertise who contribute to scoping and/or are consulted on specific matters, such as parameters of key research studies or review of the drafted guideline manuscript, in the context of their expertise or experience. Expert panelists are not guideline authors and do not participate in the literature review or vote on guideline recommendations.

guideline panel leader. However, because of the PI's prominent role in the development of the final guideline and the need for some separation between the systematic review and the guideline recommendation development processes, the project PI may not also lead the systematic review.

Conflict of Interest

The ACR requires full disclosure of all relationships, not just potential conflicts of interest, for all guideline development group (**Table 1**) members, that is, anyone who will be intellectually involved in the guideline development project. Disclosures must include companies and organizations that may be affected by the work, including but not limited to pharmaceutical, biotechnology, or other companies that manufacture or market products, or competitors of these companies. The ACR-posted "affected companies" list for each guideline is not meant to be exhaustive but to suggest companies or organizations that may constitute conflicts of interest for a particular guideline.

Individual disclosures must include any relationships within 1 year before the project start date, or relationships that exist and/or are planned during the tenure of the guideline development work (ie, through publication). The PI and the literature review team leader are also expected to avoid conflicts of interest for 1 year after publication of the guideline. The ACR requires that at least 51% of the overall guideline development group, at least 51% of the core team, at least 51% of the literature review team, and at least 51% the voting panel have no conflicts of interest.

The ACR's disclosure and conflict of interest policies are meant to deal with individuals' relationships, including conflicts, that may potentially bias how evidence is chosen, assessed, and synthesized, or bias the recommendations based on such evidence. The identification of a majority of nonconflicted individuals with the appropriate knowledge or skill set can often be challenging but is believed to be critically important to the legitimacy of the final product.

Identify Clinical Questions and Outcomes

The core team is tasked with leading the guideline development group to identify important, clinically relevant questions and outcomes. These may range from common clinical questions to areas where there is significant uncertainty (eg, what is the best second-line treatment of patients with rheumatoid arthritis after an inadequate response to methotrexate).[6] This may include traditional treatments for which there is robust evidence or new clinical dilemmas where guidance is needed because the evidence is sparse. The PICO (Population, Intervention, Comparator and Outcomes) format is used to delineate four main components necessary to construct searchable clinical questions used in evidence-based medicine.[8]

Obtain Feedback

Public feedback is solicited on the project, its scope, and clinical questions via a detailed project plan posted on the ACR Web site, which is advertised to ACR members and open to anyone to submit comments, usually for 30 days.

Conduct Systematic Review of the Literature

A systematic review of the literature, dictated to address the aforementioned PICO questions, is conducted by the literature review team. The literature review involves multiple databases (eg, Medline, Embase). This step involves an individual with database expertise, usually a medical librarian. This individual develops appropriate search strategies, in collaboration with the core team, including identification of search terms that are unique to each database. Titles and abstracts are dually screened against inclusion/exclusion criteria, followed by dual full manuscript screening.

Consider the Evidence

Evidence from the published literature is synthesized into data tables by the literature review team. Numbers of studies, study design, risk of bias, inconsistency, indirectness, imprecision, number of patients, number of control subjects, estimates of treatment effect, measures of uncertainty around the estimate of treatment effect, and quality of evidence are summarized. The evidence for each PICO question is then considered by the voting panel in the context of clinical expertise and experience, and the patient panel in the context of their experiences, values, and preferences.

The ACR uses GRADE to evaluate the evidence and make recommendations. The GRADE approach provides a transparent and systematic process for the development of recommendations that are used even when data are limited.[9,10] GRADE methodology specifies that panels reach consensus to make recommendations based on a consideration of:

- The balance of benefits and harms of the treatment options under consideration
- The quality of the evidence (ie, confidence in the effect estimates)
- Patients' values and preferences

Cost is also considered by ACR guideline development groups, when possible. A formal cost-effectiveness analysis is not conducted, rather cost is considered as one of the possible harms. If all other factors are reasonably equal but one option is considerably more costly than the other, a recommendation may favor the less costly option. Key to the recommendation is the trade-off between desirable and undesirable outcomes; recommendations require estimating the relative value patients place on the outcomes, which is achieved through patient panel input.

When transitioning from evidence to recommendations, it is important to separate judgements about the quality of evidence (confidence in estimates) from decisions about the strength of recommendations, although the two are often linked. High confidence in effect estimates does not necessarily imply strong recommendations, and conversely, strong recommendations can result from low or even very low confidence in effect estimates. For example, in patients with spinal fusion or advanced spinal osteoporosis, the 2019 guidelines for the treatment of ankylosing spondylitis and nonradiographic axial spondyloarthritis strongly recommend against treatment with spinal manipulation despite very low evidence.[11] The inability to separate considerations pertaining to quality of evidence versus strength of recommendation can lead to confusion.

The GRADE process makes a clear distinction between quality of evidence and strength of recommendations. ACR recommendations are characterized by strength, as either strong or conditional. Recommendations are based on the quality of evidence, rated as high, moderate, low, or very low (**Box 3**). Other factors, such as patient and clinician preferences and values, are also taken into consideration and are explicitly stated in the guideline recommendations.[1]

Patient Panel

A meeting of the patient panel is independently conducted just before the voting panel meeting. The patient panel is presented with the background and scope of the guideline project. They are then specifically queried on the relative importance of benefits and harms of interventions (eg, drugs, drug classes, other therapeutic options),

---

Box 3
Recommendations using the GRADE approach

- Recommendations are characterized by *strength*, as either *strong* or *conditional*
- Recommendations are based on the *quality* of evidence, rated as *high, moderate, low,* or *very low*
- Other factors, including patient and clinician preferences and values, are also taken into consideration and are explicitly stated in the guideline recommendations

including but not limited to efficacy, route of administration, and side effects, with particular attention paid to how values and preferences might differ. As part of this process, the patient panel reviews the evidence report that has been synthesized by the literature review team, with the guidance of a clinician facilitator. The participants are encouraged to consider their personal experiences relevant to the questions and judge the importance of the outcomes and give opinions on the drafted recommendation statements accordingly.[12] Two patient panelists serve on the voting panel. They represent the values and preferences of the patient panel during the voting panel's discussions and decision-making about final guideline recommendations.

Voting Panel

The voting panel reviews the evidence report. They meet face-to-face (in person or virtual) to discuss and vote on the direction and strength of the recommendations. A threshold of 70% is used to determine consensus. If 70% consensus is not achieved during an initial vote, the panel members hold additional discussions before revoting until at least 70% consensus is achieved on direction and strength. Consistent with GRADE guidance, in some instances, the voting panel may choose to provide a strong recommendation despite a low or very low quality rating of evidence.[13] In such cases, a written explanation is provided describing the reasons behind this decision with reference to GRADE guidance on the matter.[6]

Draft the Guideline Manuscript

A manuscript is drafted with a goal of balancing methodologic rigor with readability. Authors of the manuscript are encouraged to remember that consumers of the published article may vary widely, including the public, insurers, and practitioners.

Peer Review

Once the manuscript has been completed and approved by all authors, it is submitted for peer review. The manuscript is first reviewed by the ACR Guideline Subcommittee, the ACR QOC, and the ACR Board of Directors. Queries and revisions may be requested at every step. The manuscript is then submitted for journal peer review and eventual publication in ACR journals.

Guideline Publication and Dissemination

The guideline is published. Several knowledge dissemination strategies for the new guideline may be implemented. The guideline may be presented at the ACR annual scientific meeting or at an ACR-hosted town hall. Based on positive feedback from the membership on the posting of tables containing summaries of the ACR COVID-19 recommendations on the ACR Web site,[14] summary tables for all new guidelines will also be posted on the ACR Web site. The ACR supports a guideline application for mobile devices that features algorithms and the full guideline. The ACR also often produces guideline pocket cards. The guidelines are often featured in online educational Web sites, such as UpToDate.

Update of the Guideline

The evolution of medical knowledge, technology, and/or practice often occurs after publication of an ACR guideline. Updated literature searches are conducted periodically, and new literature is reviewed. The new body of evidence is re-evaluated to ascertain the need for updating or revising guidelines.

SUMMARY

Clinical practice guidelines are among the most valued products the ACR produces for its membership. The ACR places a high priority on developing methodologically rigorous, evidence-based guidelines that take into consideration the expertise and viewpoints of multiple stakeholders in a transparent fashion.

DISCLOSURE

Authors have no disclosures.

REFERENCES

1. American College of Rheumatology. Policy and procedure manual for clinical practice guidelines. American College of Rheumatology. 2015. Available at: https://www.rheumatology.org/Practice-Quality/Clinical-Support/Clinical-Practice-Guidelines. Accessed May 9, 2022.
2. Olson RM, Feldman CH. A critical look at race-based practices in rheumatology guidelines. Arthritis Care Res (Hoboken) 2021.
3. FitzGerald JD, Dalbeth N, Mikuls T, et al. 2020 American College of Rheumatology guideline for the management of gout. Arthritis Rheum 2020;72(6): 879–95.
4. Shojania KG, Sampson M, Ansari MT, et al. How quickly do systematic reviews go out of date? A survival analysis. Ann Intern Med 2007;147(4):224–33.
5. Guyatt G, Oxman AD, Akl EA, et al. GRADE guidelines: 1. introduction-GRADE evidence profiles and summary of findings tables. J Clin Epidemiol 2011;64(4): 383–94.
6. Fraenkel L, Bathon JM, England BR, et al. 2021 American College of Rheumatology guideline for the treatment of rheumatoid arthritis. Arthritis Rheum 2021; 73(7):1108–23.
7. Goodman SM, Springer BD, Chen AF, et al. 2022 American College of Rheumatology/American Association of Hip and Knee Surgeons guideline for the perioperative management of antirheumatic medication in patients with rheumatic diseases undergoing elective total hip or total knee arthroplasty. Arthritis Rheum 2022. In Press. Available at: https://www.rheumatology.org/Portals/0/Files/Perioperative-Management-Guideline-Summary.pdf. Acessed May 9, 2022.
8. Guyatt GH, Oxman AD, Kunz R, et al. GRADE guidelines: 2. framing the question and deciding on important outcomes. J Clin Epidemiol 2011;64(4):395–400.
9. Atkins D, Best D, Briss PA, et al. Grading quality of evidence and strength of recommendations. BMJ 2004;328(7454):1490.
10. Balshem H, Helfand M, Schunemann HJ, et al. GRADE guidelines: 3. rating the quality of evidence. J Clin Epidemiol 2011;64(4):401–6.
11. Ward MM, Deodhar A, Gensler LS, et al. 2019 Update of the American College of Rheumatology/Spondylitis Association of America/Spondyloarthritis Research and Treatment Network recommendations for the treatment of ankylosing spondylitis and nonradiographic axial spondyloarthritis. Arthritis Care Res (Hoboken) 2019;71(10):1285–99.
12. Fraenkel L, Miller AS, Clayton K, et al. When patients write the guidelines: patient panel recommendations for the treatment of rheumatoid arthritis. Arthritis Care Res (Hoboken) 2016;68(1):26–35.

13. Andrews JC, Schunemann HJ, Oxman AD, et al. GRADE guidelines: 15. going from evidence to recommendation-determinants of a recommendation's direction and strength. J Clin Epidemiol 2013;66(7):726–35.
14. American College of Rheumatology. COVID-19 guidance. 2022. Available at:https://www.rheumatology.org/Practice-Quality/Clinical-Support/COVID-19-Guidance. Accessed May 9, 2022.

The GRADE Method

Aydia Mayan Caplan[a,b], Liron Caplan, MD, PhD[a,b],*

KEYWORDS

- GRADE approach • Outcome assessment • Health care
- Patient outcome assessment • Evidence-based medicine • Rheumatology

KEY POINTS

- The Grades of Recommendation, Assessment, Development and Evaluation (GRADE) approach rigorously characterizes the quality of evidence from randomized clinical trials.
- The American College of Rheumatology has adapted GRADE for use in all recent clinical practice guidelines.
- Many resources are available to learn more about GRADE and the implementation of this framework.

GRADE BACKGROUND

The Grades of Recommendation, Assessment, Development and Evaluation (GRADE) approach consists of "a system for rating the quality of a body of evidence in systematic reviews and other evidence syntheses, such as health technology assessments, and guidelines and grading recommendations in health care."[1] This technique provides a common and systematic method of analyzing the medical literature in a transparent manner to convey the quality of this evidence and justify the resulting strength of recommendations in practice guidelines. The American College of Rheumatology has relied on the GRADE approach in recent clinical practice guidelines, making it the methodologic cornerstone of guideline development for rheumatologists in North America. For this reason, it is useful for rheumatologists and allied rheumatology professionals to have a working understanding of GRADE.

The original GRADE Working Group formed around 2000 as an informal group of "health care methodologists, guideline developers, clinicians, health services researchers, health economists, public health officers and other interested members."[1] The Working Group's early publications identified inconsistent methods of communicating the quality of evidence and strength of recommendations, no formal studies comparing these methods, and virtually no existing data regarding the comprehension of these systems.[2]

[a] Rocky Mountain Regional Veterans Affairs Medical Center, 1700 N. Wheeling St -111G, Aurora, CO 80045, USA; [b] University of Colorado Anschutz Medical Campus, 1775 Aurora Court – B115, Aurora, CO 80045, USA
* Corresponding author. Rheumatology Division, 1775 Aurora Court – B115, Aurora, CO 80045.
E-mail address: liron.caplan@ucdenver.edu

Rheum Dis Clin N Am 48 (2022) 589–599
https://doi.org/10.1016/j.rdc.2022.04.002
0889-857X/22/Published by Elsevier Inc.

rheumatic.theclinics.com

Since that time, GRADE has risen to become the most widely adopted tool for assessing the quality of clinical evidence, and the group has expanded to include at least 13 international GRADE centers, 6 national GRADE networks, an electronic newsletter, ongoing workshops and graduate courses on the application of GRADE, social media outlets, and online training courses. These efforts are administrated by a Guidance Group composed of 12 individuals from around the globe, as of 2020. More than 110 organizations based in at least 19 countries have used or have endorsed the GRADE approach, including the World Health Organization (WHO), US Centers for Disease Control and Prevention, and Cochrane.[3] Scores of articles related to GRADE have been published as of 2022.

INTRODUCTION TO THE BASICS OF GRADE

The essential elements of GRADE appear in **Fig. 1**. The GRADE process occurs within the context of a larger guideline development process, which is not reviewed in detail here; however, the overall process is composed of steps related to evidence synthesis and steps related to crafting recommendations. In brief, guideline developers first determine the scope of the project and then formulate structured clinical questions that posit competing management strategies.[4] These questions most frequently use the patient (or population)/intervention/comparator/outcome (PICO) format, first proposed by Richardson and colleagues; Davies has summarized this and alternative frameworks.[5] Although not included within the classic PICO format, questions frequently also specify a clinical setting and timeframe. The importance of outcomes must also be addressed explicitly, because this allows the prioritization of potentially countervailing events, such as the achievement of an efficacy end point versus an adverse drug reaction.

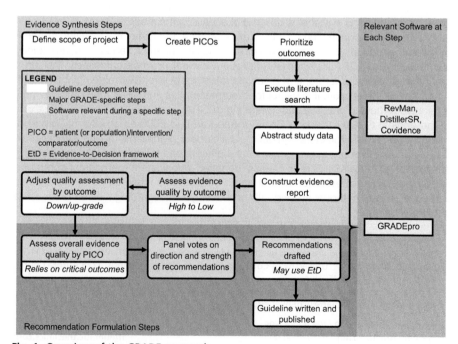

Fig. 1. Overview of the GRADE approach.

In general, American College of Rheumatology (ACR) guidelines only consider critical outcomes (those crucial for decision making), and occasionally consider important outcomes (those influencing decision making). These ACR guidelines increasingly leverage the use of patient panels to incorporate value-based assessments and perspectives during the guideline development process[6] and the GRADE method of assessing the confidence of patient preferences in qualitative studies of rheumatoid arthritis.[7]

With the clinical question (PICO) in mind, the guideline developers then execute a systematic review de novo or update an existing systematic review, to identify estimates of the outcomes associated with the competing management strategies outlined in the PICO question. It is at this stage that the GRADE process commences properly. Fundamentally, the GRADE process involves 2 principal activities:

1. Evidence synthesis: an assessment of the certainty of the compiled evidence
2. Recommendation formulation: the translation of this evidence into a recommendation, along with an estimate for the strength of the recommendation (ie, either weak or strong recommendations). Various software may facilitate some of the steps during the guideline development process, as illustrated in **Fig. 1**.

CONFIDENCE IN EVIDENCE

Confidence in evidence, also known as certainty or quality of evidence, rates a body of evidence concerning a medical intervention. Confidence in evidence may be assessed as high, moderate, low, or very low and applies to the quality across component studies, rather than the quality of individual randomized controlled trials (RCTs), per se **(Table 1)**. In general, PICOs addressed by relevant randomized trials are initially assigned high or moderate confidence in evidence, whereas those predicated on observational studies begin with a low or very low confidence in evidence.

This certainty assessment is then modulated down or up based on mitigating factors. Five such factors may downgrade the certainty rating: risk of bias, consistency of effect, imprecision, indirectness, and publication bias. The presence of any of these factors can depress the quality of the evidence by 1 level, or by 2, if the factor is very serious. In rare cases, and generally for a body of literature mainly founded on observational studies, confidence in evidence can likewise increase by 1 or 2 levels. The characteristics that can elevate the certainty assessment include the presence of a large effect size, a compelling dose-response relationship, or confounding that would have been anticipated to reduce the true effect size.[1]

Table 1		
Summary of confidence assessments		
Certainty Assessment	**Comparison of True Effect and Effect Estimated by Systematic Review Results**	**Typical Scenario Encountered by ACR Guideline Developers**
High	Estimated effects are very likely to be similar to the true effect	Multiple RCTs with results not overlapping the null effect
Moderate	Likely to be similar	A single methodologically rigorous RCT or limited number of smaller RCTs
Low	True and estimated effects may be substantially different	Indirect RCT data or a methodologically weaker study
Very low	The true and estimated effects are likely to be substantially different	No relevant RCT data or very indirectly relevant RCT data

CRITERIA THAT REDUCE CONFIDENCE IN EVIDENCE

Risk of bias refers to the degree of limitations inherent in the individual RCT within a meta-analysis. If there are methodologic deficiencies that provoke concern of bias (including subject selection, faulty randomization, inadequate blinding, imprecise outcome ascertainment, inappropriate handling of withdrawals/dropouts, and publication bias) then confidence in evidence must be downgraded. If the potential for bias is severe, raising substantial doubt in the results, confidence in evidence is downgraded by 2 levels. The assessment of bias is one of the most heavily proscribed aspects of GRADE, including advocating for the use of formal bias assessment tools and weighting of outcomes by likelihood of bias.[8–12] However, the approach adopted by the ACR during guideline development tends to rely on more qualitative assessments and a less regimented approach to the handling of bias.

Consistency of effect refers to considerable heterogeneity among results. For most comparisons in ACR guidelines, the number of studies is small, and heterogeneity is therefore considered through an informal review of study point estimates. Although the I^2 — a formal assessment of inconsistency in study outcomes — appears on virtually all outcome reports in ACR evidence summaries, it is used as the basis for determining heterogeneity only for the limited number of meta-analyses with greater numbers of component RCTs.[12,13] GRADE encourages the use of subgroup analysis and identification of the responsible modifier for instances of heterogeneity, but the ACR guideline process almost never pursues these types of detailed assessments, because the general perception is that they are unlikely to inform the resulting recommendations.[1] Of note, each outcome (whether an assessment of benefit or harm) is expressed in absolute terms for both the intervention and comparator using the same denominator on ACR Summary of Findings (SOF) tables, to allow for a direct comparison. An example of a SOF table appears as **Table 2**.

Indirectness refers to circumstances in which the most relevant evidence is unavailable, and investigators must infer assessments from related clinical scenarios. Domains of indirectness include the following:

- Population—failure to adequately represent the population of interest in the study population
- Intervention—failure to adequately represent the range of treatment dosage, or failure to adequately represent the conditions of administering the treatment
- Comparator—inclusion of a nonideal comparator group. Commonly, this manifests as the use of 2 interventional studies, each compared with similar control populations (such as a placebo group), in lieu of a head-to-head evaluation of the 2 interventions. This situation might be encountered in rheumatology for the comparison of 2 biologics—such as abatacept versus rituximab, in the management of rheumatoid arthritis, for example.
- Outcome—use of an outcome measure that must function as a surrogate for the optimal outcome measure. An example of this for the ACR might be the substitution of bone mineral density results, rather than fracture data, in guidelines for the treatment of glucocorticoid-induced osteoporosis.

Imprecision refers to width of confidence bands for the outcome of interest. The ACR follows GRADE procedures in generally reporting absolute differences for outcomes. However, ACR evidence reports make no attempt to calculate the optimal information size or review information size to determine whether the required number of participants were recruited to adequately power the analysis.[14] In most instances, the ACR guideline developers likely presume that the comparisons are underpowered.

Table 2
Example of a hypothetical American College of Rheumatology evidence report and summary of findings table (all references and data are fictional)

	Certainty Assessment						Summary of Findings				
No. of Participants (Studies) Follow-Up	Risk of Bias	Inconsistency	Indirectness	Imprecision	Publication Bias	Overall Certainty of Evidence	Study Event Rates (%)		Relative Effect (95% CI)	Anticipated Absolute Effects	
							With Placebo	With Chol_vs_NSAID		Risk With Placebo	Risk Difference With Chol_vs_NSAID
Flare counts											
3430 (4 RCTs)	Not serious	Not serious	Not serious	Not serious	None	⊕⊕⊕⊕ High	411/1297 (31.7%)	1390/2133 (65.2%)	OR 3.99 (3.27–4.88)	317 per 1000	332 more per 1000 (286 to 377 more)
CPPD radiology											
2526 (4 RCTs)	Not serious	Not serious	Not serious	Not serious	None	⊕⊕⊕⊕ High	178/881 (20.2%)	835/1645 (50.8%)	OR 4.34 (3.25–5.81)	202 per 1000	322 more per 1000 (249 to 393 more)
Chuckle											
884 (3 RCTs)	Not serious	Not serious	Not serious	Not serious	None	⊕⊕⊕○ Moderate	547	537	-	-	MD 1.32 lower (1.53 lower to 1.11 more)

(continued on next page)

Table 2
(continued)

No. of Participants (Studies) Follow-Up	Certainty Assessment						Summary of Findings				
	Risk of Bias	Inconsistency	Indirectness	Imprecision	Publication Bias	Overall Certainty of Evidence	Study Event Rates (%)		Relative Effect (95% CI)	Anticipated Absolute Effects	
							With Placebo	With Chol_vs_NSAID		Risk With Placebo	Risk Difference With Chol_vs_NSAID
Diarrhea											
2697 (2 RCTs)	Not serious	Not serious	Not serious	Not serious	None	⊕⊕⊕⊕ High	74/977 (7.6%)	452/1720 (26.3%)	OR 4.45 (3.07–6.46)	76 per 1000	191 more per 1000 (125 to 270 more)

PICO 4: In adults with active CPPD despite treatment with NSAIDs, is colchicine more effective than continuing NSAIDs in improving outcomes? [Cholchicine_vs_N-SAID for improving outcomes in adults with active CPPD despite NSAIDs (range 8–48 week; majority are 12–16 week)].

Guidance to voters: At this time, please vote with the assumption that these patients do not have comorbidities resulting in contraindications to either medication.

Summary: This PICO question was directly addressed by 4 RCTs (6 publications). One study was placebo controlled without an NSAID active comparator (Ward [1135]), and 1 prospective study was conducted without clear randomization (Feynman [2718]). Two of the studies included in this PICO question constituted new evidence not included in the 2019 guideline.

Studies directly addressing this PICO included the following NSAIDs: naproxen, sulindac, and indomethacin. Naproxen was used in 2 of the RCTs. Statistically significant between-group differences favoring colchicine were reported for most outcomes including flare counts (increased) and CPPD Radiology Assessment of Progression scores. Diarrhea was more common with colchicine. No statistically significant findings were reported for one outcome (Chuckle scores) with limited evidence.

Overall quality of evidence for all critical outcomes: High.

Abbreviations: CI, confidence interval; CPPD, calcium pyrophosphate disease; OR, odds ratio; MD, mean difference.

Bibliography {Formatted as Author [reference # in citation manager][reference # in manuscript]}: Caplan [1028][26]; Ward [1135][27]; Feynman [2718][28]; Ezra [1375][29].

Publication bias refers to exclusion of studies from publication due to their outcomes or results. The classic concern is that commercially funded studies might be more subject to publication bias. The ACR attempts to mitigate these concerns through its conflict of interest policies, although the limited number of RCTs culled for most PICOs in ACR guidelines constrains the use of quantitative evaluations of publication bias (which typically requires at least 10 RCTs).

CRITERIA THAT INCREASE CONFIDENCE IN EVIDENCE

Large effects, if consistently present in studies with no significant methodologic limitations, can raise the confidence in a body of observational studies. For a greater magnitude of effect, the confidence in evidence can still increase even despite minor shortcomings in study design. The infrequent use of observational studies for most ACR PICOs renders this largely a theoretically consideration.

Dose response refers to the presence of a gradient in responses to treatment dosages of differing amounts. This outcome strongly suggests a causal relationship between the intervention and the effect; it is unlikely that confounding variables are responsible for dose-response gradients. Therefore, the presence of a dose-response gradient can increase confidence in evidence.

Plausible confounding refers to the rare occasion in which all plausible confounding variables present in a study would plausibly reduce an effect, yet that effect is, nevertheless, evident; this increases confidence because the effect is likely stronger than what the studies seem to suggest.

For ACR-sponsored guidelines, the escalation of confidence assessments based on mitigating factors seldom occurs. In addition, it is important to note that prespecified thresholds for what constitutes a certain level of confidence do not exist. That is, the scenarios described for the ACR (see **Table 1**, column 3) are empirically observed through the process of guideline development and may not apply to other disciplines. Given the relative paucity of RCTs within rheumatology compared with other specialties, it is likely that the ACR's standard for high-certainty evidence is not compatible with more heavily studied medical disciplines.

The GRADE handbook plainly acknowledges that the GRADE approach includes an element of subjectivity in facilitating these sorts of judgements.[1] However, use of GRADE is associated with more reproducible determinations of evidence quality than assessments made without GRADE.[15]

The SOF table conveys the effect size of the intervention and comparator, the confidence in assessments as described earlier, and the rationale behind these confidence assessments. The format of SOF tables has varied slightly between ACR guidelines, with some including greater numbers of outcome measures, some including embedded citations, some reporting odds ratios and others reporting risk ratio, and varying dependence on data derived from indirect comparisons. Although these differences may seem trivial, there are reports indicating that the format of SOF tables can influence their interpretation.[16]

Translating Evidence into Recommendations and Strength of Recommendation

The procedures for converting evidence reports into recommendations are arguably more complicated and potentially more nebulous than assessing the confidence in evidence in GRADE. Ultimately, the goal is to make a recommendation that favors or counsels against the use of one therapeutic approach over another (ie, for or against the recommendation, also known as the direction of the recommendation) and to distinguish that recommendation as either strong or weak.

A group of experts, ideally representing all stakeholders affected by the resulting guidelines, considers each PICO question and votes to establish a consensus opinion. Of note, according to the convention common to ACR guideline development, PICOs are typically structured as "In population *X*, we recommend *for/against* the use of treatment *A* over treatment *B*." Thus, a vote supporting the use of treatment *A* over treatment *B* only requires a second vote to determine the strength of the recommendation. In contrast, a vote failing to support the use of treatment *A* over treatment *B* does not settle the question of whether treatment *B* should be favored over treatment *A*; this second scenario would require its own separate vote. In practice, ACR voting panels often do not consider these alternate scenarios, because they are often charged with evaluating hundreds of PICOs during a voting panel exercise.

Once the direction of a PICO is established, the voting panel considers the strength of the recommendation. Recommendations are stronger when the benefits of treatment clearly outweigh the harms, whether those be health risks, inconveniences, or financial costs (**Table 3**). Recommendations should take into account the confidence of evidence, as well as factors such as physical effects of the treatment, cost or feasibility, equity, as well as the acceptability and feasibility of the therapeutic options. A strong recommendation implies that when informed of the treatment, most patients will select to undergo it; a weak recommendation implies that the choice of whether to undergo a treatment will reflect individual patients' values and preferences. The latter type demands a more involved decision-making process. The designation of a recommendation as either strong or weak is not without consequence: strongly rated guidelines are statistically more likely to produce changes in public policy.[17]

Although some organizations and research groups use formal Evidence-to-Decision frameworks to guide and document the translation of evidence into discreet recommendations, the ACR generally does not follow this approach.[1] Instead, a more informal strategy is used. The ACR has used various methods of visually depicting

Table 3 Strong versus conditional recommendations		
	Category of Recommendation	
Characteristic	**Weak/Conditional**	**Strong**
Balance of benefits and harms	Less clear balance	More clearly favors either benefits or harms
Generalizability of recommendation	Clinician applies to only a portion of patients	Clinician applies to most patients with fewer exceptions
Use of shared decision making	Shared decision making is the focus of the clinical visit	Implementation of the decision in the focus of the visit
Mitigating considerations	Frequently present	Less frequently present
Patient preferences	A substantial number of patients may not agree on best course of action	More universal acceptance of a single course of action among well-informed patients
Policy implications	Too much variation in opinion to justify use as a quality indicator	Substantial consensus in opinion to justify use as a quality indicator

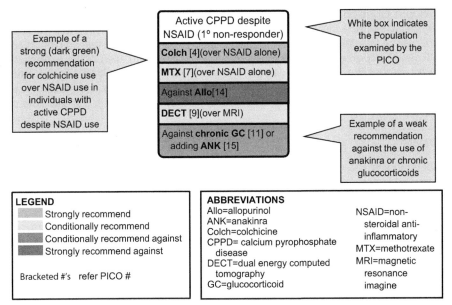

Fig. 2. Color-coded representation of direction and strength of recommendations in hypothetical ACR guideline for calcium pyrophosphate disease (no such guideline currently exists).

recommendations over the years, including tables and flowcharts. One such color-coded approach appears in **Fig. 2**.

ONLINE TOOLS AND RESOURCES

The production of guidelines using the GRADE approach requires a certain degree of expertise and reliance on fairly specialized tools, including online training resources, expository articles related to GRADE, as well as digital tools to facilitate data management and for recording the various assessments mentioned earlier (see **Fig. 1**).

The primary authority for the GRADE approach is the freely available GRADE handbook.[1] This document provides a fairly succinct summary of GRADE, but has not been revised since 2013. GRADE training materials are also available in other forms, including GRADE online training modules hosted by the Cochrane collaboration (https://training.cochrane.org/grade-approach). This digital resource includes slideshows, webinars, self-paced learning modules, and articles.

Similarly, the WHO has assembled its own repository of more than 20 YouTube videos describing various aspects of GRADE. This video library is located at https://www.youtube.com/c/MacGRADECentre with each video running anywhere from 3 to 33 minutes in duration.

In addition, the *Journal of Clinical Epidemiology* has published an extensive collection of more than 30 articles that provide an in-depth and comprehensive understanding of all aspects of the GRADE approach (https://www.jclinepi.com/content/jce-GRADE-Series).

Several software tools ease the early synthesis steps of guideline development, including tools to screen reference titles, abstracts, and manuscripts (DistillerSR and Covidence), and tools to perform meta-analyses (Review Manager, ie, RevMan). Last, the GRADE Working Group, in partnership with McMaster University, has developed GRADEpro Guideline Development Tool (GRADEpro GDT). This is the primary online software that assists in creating SOF tables for literature reviews. The software may be installed as a stand-alone application or online to facilitate collaboration. Data can be imported directly from ReviewManager (RevMan), the Cochrane application for conducting systematic literature reviews. As of 2022, GRADEpro has been used by more than 95,000 users and remains free of charge for groups of up to 3 researchers. The tool itself, as well as instruction videos for using it, are available at www.gradepro.org.

SUMMARY

Understanding the GRADE approach is of critical importance for guideline developers and is potentially useful to health care providers, who should understand the strengths and limitations of this methodologic approach underpinning the most recent ACR clinical practice guidelines. Understanding the approach is also of use to policymakers, who need some knowledge of the method used to formulate the evidence required for health care policy decisions. Both groups should recognize the modifications necessary to adapt this framework to the needs of the rheumatology community.

CLINICS CARE POINTS

- As clinicians employ American College of Rheumatology guidelines, they can recognize elements of the GRADE approach–such the strength of evidence–and include these elements in their decisionmaking.
- The GRADE approach can furnish health care providers with a systematic framework that facilitates the use of evidence while making choices with their patients.

DISCLOSURE

The author has nothing to disclose. Dr L. Caplan's time was supported in part by the Rocky Mountain Regional Veterans Affairs Medical Center. The views expressed in this article are those of the authors and do not necessarily reflect the position or policy of the Department of Veterans Affairs. The authors wish to acknowledge Amy Turner at the American College of Rheumatology, for her feedback and insight.

REFERENCES

1. Schünemann, Holger J, Brożek J, Guyatt G, et al. GRADE handbook. 2013. Available at: https://gdt.gradepro.org/app/handbook/handbook.html. Accessed April 2, 2022.
2. Schünemann HJ, Best D, Vist G, et al. Letters, numbers, symbols and words: how to communicate grades of evidence and recommendations. Can Med Assoc J 2003;169:677. LP – 680. Available at: http://www.cmaj.ca/content/169/7/677. abstract. Accessed April 2, 2022.
3. The GRADE Working Group. GRADE. 2022. Available at: https://www.gradeworkinggroup.org/. Accessed April 2, 2022.
4. Guyatt GH, Oxman AD, Kunz R, et al. GRADE guidelines: 2. Framing the question and deciding on important outcomes. J Clin Epidemiol 2011;64:395–400.

5. Davies KS. Formulating the evidence based practice question: a review of the frameworks. Evid Based Libr Inf Pract 2011;6:75–80.

6. Fraenkel L, Miller AS, Clayton K, et al. When patients write the guidelines: patient panel recommendations for the treatment of rheumatoid arthritis. Arthritis Care Res 2016;68:26–35.

7. Harrison M, Marra C, Shojania K, et al. Societal preferences for rheumatoid arthritis treatments: evidence from a discrete choice experiment. Rheumatology 2015;54:1816–25. https://doi.org/10.1093/rheumatology/kev113. Available at:.

8. Guyatt GH, Oxman AD, Vist G, et al. GRADE guidelines: 4. Rating the quality of evidence–study limitations (risk of bias). J Clin Epidemiol 2011;64:407–15. https://doi.org/10.1016/j.jclinepi.2010.07.017. Available at:.

9. Guyatt GH, Oxman AD, Montori V, et al. GRADE guidelines: 5. Rating the quality of evidence–publication bias. J Clin Epidemiol 2011;64:1277–82. https://doi.org/10.1016/j.jclinepi.2011.01.011. Available at:.

10. Guyatt GH, Ebrahim S, Alonso-Coello P, et al. GRADE guidelines 17: assessing the risk of bias associated with missing participant outcome data in a body of evidence. J Clin Epidemiol 2017;87:14–22. https://doi.org/10.1016/j.jclinepi.2017.05.005. Available at:.

11. Zhang Y, Alonso-Coello P, Guyatt GH, et al. GRADE Guidelines: 19. Assessing the certainty of evidence in the importance of outcomes or values and preferences—Risk of bias and indirectness. J Clin Epidemiol 2019;111:94–104. https://doi.org/10.1016/j.jclinepi.2018.01.013. Available at:.

12. Schünemann HJ, Mustafa RA, Brozek J, et al. GRADE guidelines: 21 part 2. Test accuracy: inconsistency, imprecision, publication bias, and other domains for rating the certainty of evidence and presenting it in evidence profiles and summary of findings tables. J Clin Epidemiol 2020;122:142–52. https://doi.org/10.1016/j.jclinepi.2019.12.021. Available at:.

13. Guyatt GH, Oxman AD, Kunz R, et al. GRADE guidelines: 7. Rating the quality of evidence–inconsistency. J Clin Epidemiol 2011;64:1294–302. https://doi.org/10.1016/j.jclinepi.2011.03.017. Available at:.

14. Guyatt GH, Oxman AD, Kunz R, et al. GRADE guidelines 6. Rating the quality of evidence–imprecision. J Clin Epidemiol 2011;64:1283–93. https://doi.org/10.1016/j.jclinepi.2011.01.012. Available at:.

15. Mustafa RA, Santesso N, Brozek J, et al. The GRADE approach is reproducible in assessing the quality of evidence of quantitative evidence syntheses. J Clin Epidemiol 2013;66:735–6.

16. Carrasco-Labra A, Brignardello-Petersen R, Santesso N, et al. Improving GRADE evidence tables part 1: a randomized trial shows improved understanding of content in summary of findings tables with a new format. J Clin Epidemiol 2016;74:7–18. https://doi.org/10.1016/j.jclinepi.2015.12.007. Available at:.

17. Nasser SMU, Cooke G, Kranzer K, et al. Strength of recommendations in WHO guidelines using GRADE was associated with uptake in national policy. J Clin Epidemiol 2015;68:703–7.

Taxonomy of Quality of Care Indicators

Tracing the Path from Clinical Practice Guidelines to Quality Measurement and Beyond

Elizabeth Wahl, MD, MAS[a,b], Una E. Makris, MD, MSc[c],
Lisa G. Suter, MD[d,e,*]

KEYWORDS

- Quality • Measurement • Guidelines • Value • Outcomes

KEY POINTS

- Quality measures help improve care quality by directing quality improvement activities, incentivizing best practices, and assisting patients in selecting health care providers.
- The different types of quality measures can be optimally designed to best serve their intended use while minimizing unintended results.
- Quality measures can be used for rapid cycle quality improvement or for high-stakes programs, such as pay-for-reporting and pay-for-performance programs.

BACKGROUND AND DEFINITIONS

Clinical practice guidelines (CPGs) summarize the best available evidence to create standards for optimizing patient care; quality measures (QMs) quantify and track processes and outcomes of care meaningful to patients and clinicians. QMs are standards of performance in health care. Often the term is used interchangeably with quality indicators (QIs); for example, the Agency for Healthcare Research and Quality uses QIs, whereas the Centers for Medicare and Medicaid Services (CMS) uses QM. Herein, the authors use QM. Together, QMs and CPGs support the delivery of

[a] Department of Medicine, Division of Rheumatology, University of Washington; [b] VA Puget Sound Healthcare System, 1660 South Columbian Way, S-111 ARTH, Seattle, WA 98108, USA; [c] VA North Texas Health System, 5323 Harry Hines Boulevard, Suite 9169, Dallas, TX 775390-9169, USA; [d] Yale School of Medicine, PO Box 208031, 300 Cedar Street, New Haven, CT 06520, USA; [e] Connecticut Veterans Health Administration, 950 Campbell Avenue, West Haven, CT 06516, USA
* Corresponding author. Yale School of Medicine, PO Box 208031, 300 Cedar Street, New Haven, CT 06520.
E-mail address: lisa.suter@yale.edu
Twitter: @WahlMD (E.W.); @UnaMakris (U.E.M.)

Rheum Dis Clin N Am 48 (2022) 601–615
https://doi.org/10.1016/j.rdc.2022.03.004
0889-857X/22/Published by Elsevier Inc.

effective, evidence-based, high-quality care. The authors establish a framework for learners to understand the relevance, development, and validation of QMs in rheumatology, touching on their relationship to guidelines and appropriate use criteria (AUC). They also describe measure implementation and reflect on associated challenges and opportunities.

Why Measure Quality?

High-quality care should not only be safe, effective, patient-centered, timely, efficient, and equitable, but also must go beyond this to improve the patient experience of care and the health of populations, while reducing the per-capita cost. This framework is known as the Triple Aim. To improve the performance of the US health care system, 3 components are needed: "improving the experience of care, improving the health of populations, and reducing per capita costs of health care."[1] Addressing clinician burnout and advancing health equity are proposed additional guideposts.[2,3] Advancing the Triple Aim requires meaningful measurement to leverage data and relationships to drive a learning health care system.

Health care disparities, high rates of medical error, and gaps in adherence to minimum care standards produce a focus on measuring quality of care.[4,5] Significant variation in care and outcomes exists by geographic region, physician specialty, and patient demographics (eg, race and ethnicity) across rheumatologic conditions,[6] including rheumatoid arthritis (RA),[7–9] gout,[10] osteoarthritis,[11] osteoporosis,[12] and lupus.[13] Patient outcomes improve with early diagnosis and treatment.[14–18] Outcomes are enhanced by adherence to methodologically rigorous, evidence-based CPGs.[19,20] An "evidence-practice" gap often results, creating opportunities to improve implementation of guideline-concordant care.[21,22]

Quality measurement then builds on this foundation to illuminate disparities in care, highlight opportunities for improvement, and promote best practice care (**Fig. 1**).[23,24] Stakeholders, including health care plans, employers, government agencies, professional societies, and the public, are invested in quality measurement and reporting to prioritize opportunities for improvement. Patients may use QMs to select health care clinicians or systems, or to monitor their own outcomes. Clinicians may use QMs to modify practice behaviors, optimize patient outcomes, reduce disparities, or reduce wasted expenditures to improve value. Payers may use QMs to guide reimbursement and resource allocation.

What Is a Quality Measure?

QMs are tools that help quantify health care processes, outcomes, patient perceptions, and organizational structures and systems associated with high-quality health care.[25] QMs are often categorized as structure, process, and outcome (**Fig. 2**).[26,27] Although the thinking has evolved over time, this model is still relevant. Measures can be further categorized by their application, such as balancing measures.

Structure QMs describe innate characteristics of clinicians and health care systems and whether they have the basic components to provide health care. Examples include the number of rheumatologists or unfilled positions in a clinic or the training and certification of staff. Structure QMs provide an important foundation for provision of high-quality care, but they are insufficient to guarantee it.

Process QMs reflect what clinicians do when delivering care: is a disease activity measure recorded at each clinic visit for patients with RA? Are prescreening laboratory tests and vaccinations completed before initiation of biologic therapy? Although process QMs do not always translate to improved patient outcomes, they offer a roadmap

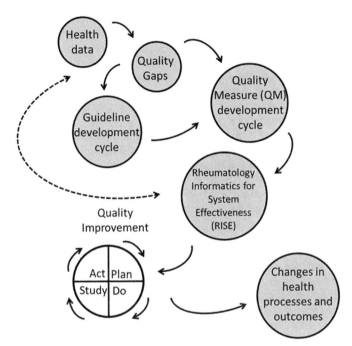

Fig. 1. Interrelationship of practice guidelines, quality measurements, and quality improvement. Quality gaps are identified through health data assessment. Evidence-based CPGs inform best practice care, which informs QM development, which can support rapid cycle quality improvement. Registries, such as the ACR's RISE registry, are important for this process, as they provide data demonstrating quality gaps, a robust environment for measure development and testing, and support QM implementation.

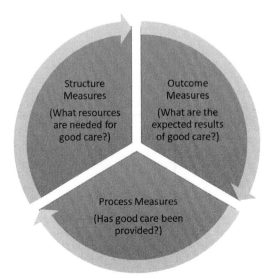

Fig. 2. Donabedian's model for measuring quality of care. Structure measures capture the foundational resources needed to provide health care. Process measures provide a roadmap for good care. Outcome measures capture what we expect good care to yield.

to high-quality care informed by CPGs. Most QMs in use, including in rheumatology, are process measures, as outcome QMs are challenging to develop and implement.[28]

Outcome QMs reflect the impact of health care on patients. Examples include the proportion of patients with RA in sustained clinical remission or the proportion of patients with knee osteoarthritis experiencing improved mobility and decreased pain following knee replacement. Although outcome measures capture what is meaningful to patients, in isolation they do not help explain the system that created them, nor do they direct how to improve poor outcomes.

Outcome QMs should be distinguished from outcome measures, such as those defined and promoted by the Outcome Measures in Rheumatology (OMERACT) Initiative. OMERACT develops and validates standardized instruments to collect meaningful patient outcomes, such as disease activity, functional status, quality of life, and organ damage.[29] These assessments are often used as target endpoints in clinical trials, and they are important QM components; a QM evaluating RA functional status improvement might use the Patient-Reported Outcomes Measurement Information System Physical Function outcome measure to capture functional status.[30]

Balancing measures are QMs that may have limited individual utility but provide critical surveillance to ensure improvement in one area does not adversely impact another area. They can assess structures, processes, and outcomes. For example, a QM evaluating the proportion of patients with RA achieving low disease activity could unintentionally encourage clinicians to use excessive glucocorticoids to achieve lower disease activity. Steroids can decrease disease activity, but may also produce higher rates of infection, hospitalization, or bone loss. Simultaneously measuring a patient's cumulative steroid exposure, hospitalization or infection rates, and/or osteoporotic fractures could all serve as balancing measures for such a QM.

What Are the Components of a Quality Measure?

QM components include a title/description of the measure, the health care structure, process, or outcome being measured (numerator), the population being measured (denominator or cohort), the relevant time period, and to whom the measure is attributed (**Fig. 3**).[31]

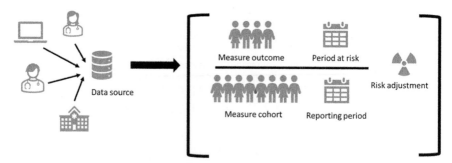

Measure outcome   Period at risk

Data source   Risk adjustment

Measure cohort   Reporting period

Fig. 3. Anatomy of a QM. QMs use data from claims, clinical registries, surveys, and EHR. The measure cohort includes the patients for whom the outcome is measured. The measure outcome is recorded over a distinct period called the reporting period; the longer the time covered, the more precise but less actionable the output. The measure outcome captures the clinical outcomes, patient experience, or other results of care that are the focus of the measure. Risk adjustment adjusts the outcomes of different clinicians according to the risk level of the patients on which they are being measured to promote more accurate comparisons between groups.

For example, an electronic Clinical Quality Measure (eCQM) for gout is "the proportion of patients ages $\geq$18 years with a diagnosis of gout treated with urate lowering therapy (ULT) for at least 12 months, whose most recent serum uric acid (sUA) result is <6.0 mg/dL."[32] This is a clinician-level process measure encouraging guideline-concordant, treat-to-target care for gout patients. The numerator is the proportion of patients with an sUA less than 6.0; the denominator includes a clinician's adult gout patients $\geq$18 years treated with ULT for at least 12 months, except for patients with a history of solid organ transplant, use of tacrolimus, or cyclosporine, or estimated glomerular filtration rate level less than 30 mL/min or stage 4 or greater chronic kidney disease or end-stage renal disease in the measurement year or year prior; the measure is attributed to clinicians, and the relevant time period is 1 year.·

How Are Quality Measures Different from Clinical Practice Guidelines and Appropriate Use Criteria?

QMs are often developed from CPGs. Although QMs and CPGs share the goal of standardizing and improving patient care and outcomes, they are distinct (**Table 1**). CPGs provide specific recommendations around the quality of evidence supporting diagnostic, therapeutic, and management decisions for a given condition.[33,34] CPGs are developed based on evidence as well as other factors, such as clinical experience and expertise, patient values and preferences, and cost. Ideally, both QMs and CPGs are developed using high-quality data by expert panels with diverse stakeholder representation without conflicts of interest and undergo a consensus-based iterative assessment of the evidence, such as the modified RAND Appropriateness Method[35] (see articles "ACR policies and procedures for guideline development" and "The GRADE method"). In practice, CPGs may include some recommendations based solely on expert input owing to the absence of robust, relevant evidence, and there may be value in tracking outcome QMs like fatigue in systemic lupus erythematosus, despite limited evidence defining how to reduce this symptom.

Appropriate Use Criteria (AUC) are a type of guideline intended to define appropriateness (that is, when expected benefits substantially exceed expected risks) of procedures or other interventions in distinct patient groups based on the best available evidence.[36,37] AUC are useful when there is significant variation in care, including overuse or underuse, and in high-cost (surgical procedures, diagnostic radiology) or limited resource settings. Unlike CPGs, AUC are often linked to decision support tools and guide care decisions in an individual patient by outlining recommended care for patients in a specific clinical situation.[36] The 2014 Protecting Access to Medicare Act passed by Congress mandates AUC development in radiology, cardiology, and orthopedics to improve quality of care and reduce unnecessary testing. To date, the American College of Rheumatology (ACR) has prioritized CPGs and improving access for expensive and novel therapeutics over AUC.

How Are Quality Measures Developed?

Process quality measures
The ACR methodology for process eCQM development consists of concept development and testing.[38] An interdisciplinary expert panel, including patients, is convened that develops candidate metrics using one or more CPG. The panel rates the evidence supporting each concept, relevant psychometric properties, and feasibility. Measure concepts are finalized as IF/THEN/BECAUSE statements (**Fig. 4**). For example, IF a patient with gout is initiated on ULT, THEN anti-inflammatory prophylaxis should be used concomitantly consisting of low-dose colchicine, nonsteroidal anti-inflammatory drug, or glucocorticoid, BECAUSE concomitant use of prophylaxis

Table 1
Comparing and contrasting clinical practice guidelines and quality measures

	Clinical Practice Guideline	Quality Measure
Purpose	Summarize best available evidence to establish standards for high-quality care Example: Improve care of patients with gout by establishing best practices for gout treatment	Quantify and track effectiveness and outcomes; reward good care and/or penalize poor care; select optimal providers/facilities Example: Enable eligible clinicians to evaluate their health care practices and compare them with best practices
Format	Narrative: For a given clinical scenario, state strength of recommendation and report quality of evidence Example: For all patients taking ULT, the authors strongly recommend continuing ULT to achieve and maintain an SUA target of <6.0mg/dL over no target[61]	For process measures, a proportion of a defined eligible population meeting a particular minimally acceptable metric over a defined period For outcome quality measures, observed vs expected patient-level outcome of interest in defined eligible population over a defined period accounting for patient case mix Example: ACR's proportion of patients ages ≥18 y with a diagnosis of gout treated with ULT for at least 12 mo, whose most recent sUA result is <6.0 mg/dL[32] Example: Risk-adjusted proportion of RA patients in remission or low disease activity
Used by	Clinicians and, increasingly, patients Examples: Clinicians use guidelines to inform their treatment choices for patients; patients can use published guidelines to educate themselves and communicate with their health care clinician, as part of shared decision making	Clinicians, health care systems; quality reporting, accreditation, payment programs, patients Examples: Clinicians can audit their own clinical practice by tracking their measure results; CMS can provide monetary incentive payments or penalties; patients might use the public information provided by CMS[53] or other quality rating organizations like ProPublica to choose a clinician

reduces the risk of gout flares.[32] These concepts are operationalized as process QMs by defining the numerator, denominator, attribution, and relevant risk period (see **Fig. 3**). Detailed specifications are then tested across multiple settings, including ensuring the results are reliably and feasibly captured, and represent a validated assessment of quality.[38–42] Importantly, measures should be feasible to collect and implement.[43,44] Feasibility requires careful evaluation of the data source or sources used for measure calculation, with a goal of minimizing clinician and patient burden while maximizing information accuracy, reproducibility, and validity.[45]

Many QMs intended for high-stakes use, such as public reporting or payment, are submitted to the National Quality Forum (NQF) for vetting by experts. NQF is a consensus-based not-for-profit, nonpartisan, membership-based organization that evaluates and endorses QMs.[39] The ACR has 7 measures that are either NQF

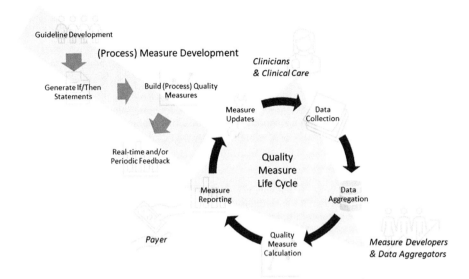

Fig. 4. Interrelationship of QM development and life cycle with clinicians, payers, and other health care stakeholders. Measure development is a stakeholder-driven, stepwise process, starting from clinical evidence, through defining measure specifications, and testing the measure for scientific acceptability and feasibility. QMs then enter an implementation life cycle, where data are collected for public or confidential measure reporting. Feedback from clinical experience with the measures and/or evolving evidence and clinical practice informs regular measure updates.

endorsed or approved for trial use; 3 of these measures (or similar versions stewarded by the ACR) are part of the Center for Medicare and Medicaid Services (CMS) Quality Payment Program (QPP) Merit-Based Incentive Payment System (MIPS), in addition to a measure assessing glucocorticoid management (**Box 1**). NQF evaluates measures for endorsement using the following 4 criteria:

- Importance
- Scientific acceptability, including producing reproducible, valid results
- Usability and relevance to optimal care
- Feasibility with minimal patient and provider burden

Regardless of QM type (structure, process, outcome), these criteria are critical pillars for ensuring QMs can advance health care quality without unintended consequences.

Outcome quality measures

Outcome QMs capture positive or negative health care outcomes. Positive outcomes assess desirable health care outcomes, including reduction in pain, improvement in function, and sustained clinical remission. Negative outcomes include unintended consequences of health care, such as adverse drug events, complications, hospitalization, disability, and death. Outcome QMs leverage outcome assessments (also called outcome measures, confusingly), such as those vetted by OMERACT, to define the outcome the measure is intended to assess. Outcome QMs are developed in a similar manner to process QMs; they are informed by high-quality evidence, evaluated by clinical and technical experts, and assessed to ensure they meet the same NQF

Box 1
Rheumatology quality measures endorsed by the National Quality Forum or approved for trial use

Gout measures
- Gout: Serum urate target (NQF#2549e: Approved for eMeasure Trial use)—Percentage of patients aged 18 years and older with a diagnosis of gout treated with ULT for at least 12 months, whose most recent serum urate result is less than 6.0 mg/dL.
- Gout: ULT therapy (NQF2550e: Approved for eMeasure Trial use)—Percentage of patients aged 18 years and older with a diagnosis of gout and either tophus/tophi or at least 2 gout flares (attacks) in the past year who have a serum urate level greater than 6.0 mg/dL, who are prescribed ULT.

Rheumatoid arthritis measures
- Rheumatoid Arthritis: Assessment of Diseases Activity (NQF#2523: Endorsed; QPP#177: 2021 MIPS program)—Percentage of patients 18 years and older with a diagnosis of RA and $\geq$ 50% of total number outpatient RA encounters in the measurement year with assessment of disease activity using standardized measure.
- Rheumatoid Arthritis: Disease Modifying Anti-Rheumatic Drug (DMARD) Therapy (NQF2525: Approved for eMeasure Trial Use)—Percentage of patients 18 years and older with a diagnosis of RA who are newly prescribed disease-modifying antirheumatic drug (DMARD) therapy within 12 months.
- Rheumatoid Arthritis: Patient-Reported Functional Status Assessment (NQF#2524e: Endorsed; variation QPP#178: 2021 MIPS program)—Percentage of patients 18 years and older with a diagnosis of RA for whom a functional status assessment was performed at least once during the measurement period.
- Rheumatoid Arthritis: Tuberculosis Screening (NQF#2522: Approved for eMeasure Trial Use; variation QPP#176: 2021 MIPS program)—Percentage of patients 18 years and older with a diagnosis of RA who have documentation of a tuberculosis screening performed within 6 months before receiving a first course of therapy using a biologic DMARD.
- Rheumatoid Arthritis: Glucocorticoid Management (QPP#180: 2021 MIPS Program)—Percentage of patients 18 years and older with a diagnosis of RA who have been assessed for glucocorticoid use and, for those on prolonged doses of prednisone greater than 5 mg daily (or equivalent) with improvement or no change in disease activity, documentation of glucocorticoid management plan within 12 months.

---

criteria of importance, scientific acceptability, usability, and feasibility. However, unlike processes of care, outcomes vary based on the health status of the patient.[46] Therefore, to compare clinicians fairly, outcome QMs must account for differences in patient case mix. For example, differences in the number of older, frail patients should be accounted for so that a clinician who sees mostly older patients would not be penalized in rating the QM.

QMs use risk adjustment to account for case mix differences. Patient risk factors, such as age, comorbidities, disease severity, and disease duration, can be added to a multivariable regression model to control for their contribution to the outcome of interest. These risk factors allow one to estimate the expected likelihood of that patient achieving an outcome. The expected outcomes for a clinician's patients can then be compared with the observed outcomes for those patients. The magnitude of residual differences in outcomes then theoretically represents that provider's quality.

There is an ongoing debate about how to account for social determinants of health (SDOH) in QMs.[47] Clinicians, measure developers, and payers agree that one goal of quality measurement is to reduce health care disparities between patients with and without social risk factors, including race/ethnicity (which are proxy indicators for exposure to systemic racism), socioeconomic status, transportation access, literacy, and other SDOH. A complete review of this topic is not feasible, but there are key points worth noting. Briefly, it is important to consider the intended purpose of the QM when considering how to account for SDOH. For example, if the goal is to illuminate disparities between patients of different races and/or ethnicities, one might examine measured results stratified by patient race and/or ethnicity. Notably, including race as a variable in the risk model would not provide the desired result of clearly identifying disparities and might even reinforce them. If black patients with RA are less likely to achieve remission than white patients in a QM assessing the risk-adjusted proportion of a rheumatologist's patients with RA in remission, then the risk model will expect black patients with RA to have lower (worse) rates of remission. Thus, when a clinician's black patients have worse outcomes than their white patients, the QM will see this as the clinician having performed as expected. If this same clinicians' black patients with RA do better than the average clinician's black patients with RA, then this clinician will have better than average QM performance, even if their black patients with RA are still doing worse than their white patients. This might be reasonable in some circumstances to ensure clinicians caring for underserved populations (for example, in a safety-net setting) are not unduly penalized, as such clinicians might need greater resources to provide optimal care for such populations. However, it does not help clinicians understand that their black patients have worse outcomes than their white patients nor does it help us move toward greater health equity by incentivizing equal outcomes for black and white patients.

Another approach might be to instead account for race when determining payment based on the QM result. The CMS has implemented this approach in its Hospital Readmission Reduction Program, where readmission measure risk models do not include SDOH; rather, hospitals are stratified by their proportion of dual-eligible patients (that is, enrolled in both Medicare and Medicaid, a common proxy for socioeconomic status) for payment determination. This ensures hospitals caring for high proportions of patients with social risk are compared with similar hospitals. The ACR is actively expanding its prioritizing of health equity across its work, including quality measurement.

Outcome QMs are important because they represent patient-centered outcomes.[48] Ensuring the outcomes measured are both important to patients and can be influenced by high-quality care requires close collaboration between patients, clinicians, and measure developers to find an acceptable intersection of importance and feasibility. This collaboration is important, as QMs are increasingly used for high-stakes applications, including clinician payment. Outcome QMs are a priority for CMS and other payers, as they allow more meaningful value-based payment, where providers are paid for the quality, not the quantity, of care they provide. However, process QMs will always be valuable because they provide a roadmap to achieve optimal outcomes.

How Are Quality Measures Implemented and Used?

Once a QM is developed, it can be implemented for a variety of uses. QMs are used in quality reporting, accreditation, payment programs, and/or locally for rapid-cycle quality improvement. They may measure quality provided by individuals, by health care systems, or within geographic regions. Most QMs used in payment or reporting programs are stewarded to ensure the measures are updated regularly to account for changes in clinical practice and data standards. This creates a QM life cycle (see **Fig. 4**) that allows measures to stay scientifically rigorous and clinically valid. CMS has created criteria for "sunsetting" (retiring) measures once they no longer offer opportunity for improvement. Most often these identify measures that are "topped out," meaning that most or all reporting entities have perfect (or nearly perfect) scores, and this performance pattern has not changed, suggesting there is little to no room for improvement.

The ACR develops QMs for use by its members and US rheumatologists. The ACR Rheumatology Informatics System for Effectiveness (RISE) registry is a Qualified Clinical Data Registry approved by CMS to develop and submit QMs to CMS on behalf of clinicians. The RISE registry is electronic health record (EHR) enabled and contains HIPAA-compliant data for more than 1000 rheumatology clinicians and 2.4 million patients. It is a powerful data set for research, QM development, and improving outcomes for patients with rheumatology.[49,50] The ACR develops and implements QMs in RISE for its members, providing detailed dashboards on clinician performance to support quality improvement and value-based payment. Measure implementation involves the ACR updating its registry to reflect the measure specifications, which dictate what data elements and information are pulled (or pushed) from a participant's EHR for measure calculations.

After an initial onboarding phase to ensure the registry receives accurate data from the clinician, practice, or system, the data exchange is automated to minimize burden. For example, all disease activity assessments for a practice's patients with RA will be pulled into the registry along with any relevant metadata, such as encounter date and clinician name. The registry then uses these data to calculate a measure result for each practice and/or individual clinician. These results are sent to clinicians for review and to inform quality improvement efforts and, if applicable, to CMS as part of its measurement programs (see later discussion).[51,52] Patients may use QMs to select clinicians or make decisions about their care, or to track their own progress.[53,54] Clinicians may use QMs to reduce waste via LEAN Methodology process improvement, to optimize patient outcomes, and/or to reduce disparities in their practice. Payers may use QMs to guide reimbursement and resource allocation, as in value-based payment programs.

Physician payment changed in 2015, when the Medicare Access and CHIP Reauthorization Act of 2015 (MACRA) replaced the Sustainable Growth Rate law. MACRA created the QPP, which offers 2 pathways for payment: the Merit-based Incentive Payment System (MIPS) and Advanced Alternative Payment Models (APMs).[55] The APM pathway is a value-based payment program, but most rheumatologists participate in MIPS, as there are currently no rheumatology-specific APMs in QPP. MIPS calculates a 0- to 100-point score for each eligible clinician or clinician group (practice) that combines quality, cost, practice improvement activities, and use of certified EHR technology to support and promote the electronic exchange of health information; in 2021, quality measurement represented 40% of one's MIPS score. This final MIPS score then determines a clinician's payment adjustment for Part B–covered professional services, which can be negative (penalty), neutral, or positive (bonus).

CMS' 2022 Physician Fee Schedule final rule, which dictates payment for physicians through the QPP, finalized several new MIPS Value Pathways (MVPs), including a Rheumatology MVP submitted by the ACR. MVPs are intended to define the set of QMs reported within a clinical specialty to allow for more informative performance comparisons.[56] Optimal QM use requires close alignment of measure development and the measure life cycle (see **Fig. 4**).

WHAT ARE SOME OF THE CHALLENGES WITH QUALITY MEASUREMENT?

It is important to remember is that no QM is perfect. Good QMs effectively serve the purpose for which they were designed.[57] They balance the burden of data collection and reporting with capturing the information needed to accurately measure the health care structure, process, or outcome of interest. A QM intended for local quality improvement activities might focus on rapid cycle assessment of disease activity in patients with RA. As such, this QM might be reported monthly to help clinicians improve assessment and documentation of disease activity. It can provide important trend information but may lead to overweighting of small monthly changes owing to the small sample size and instability of results. In contrast, a QM intended for use in a pay-for-performance program might require larger sample sizes and a longer period of data collection to ensure reliable results.

With the increase of value-based care, QMs and other tools for improving quality, like best practice alerts, have proliferated. Some warn of clinician and patient burnout owing to an excess of measures distracting from the clinician-patient relationship.[58] Many QMs require clinicians and/or patients complete lengthy surveys, manually abstract information from medical records, and/or manually input data so the data are available in the EHR. The 2021 Consumer Assessment of Healthcare Providers and Systems (CAHPS) for MIPS survey asks patients to respond to 59 distinct questions about their experience of care.[59] This may explain its low response rate, averaging around 30% or lower.

Ideal QMs also address potential unintended consequences, by either thoughtful design, use of balancing measures, or implementing the QM to avoid or reduce the likelihood of unintended consequences. Increasing focus on health equity adds another critical layer of complexity to quality measurement. A recent opinion piece highlighted the challenges of accounting for implicit bias and the effects of systemic racism in patient satisfaction QMs, such as CAHPS.[60]

Where Are Quality Measures Going?

Although these challenges seem daunting, there are reasons for optimism. Clinicians and EHR vendors are working to leverage the millions of clinical data points generated during routine clinical care to improve health care quality. Many hospitals have sophisticated risk assessment tools that analyze trends and patterns in vital signs, laboratory tests, and other clinical data to warn of impending adverse events, such as readmissions, hospital-acquired infections, or the need for ventilatory support or escalated care. These approaches use data within a clinician's health care system. The Office of the National Coordinator for Health Information Technology and CMS are united in establishing shared data standards for health care data to allow for learning and coordinated care across settings and clinicians. CMS has prioritized data interoperability as a key component of future quality measurement. Leveraging data already generated through clinical care could greatly reduce the burden of QM data collection and reporting. QMs are a critical part of supporting best practices and will remain important for decades to come.

RESOURCES

The American College of Rheumatology (ACR) Guideline and Criteria app (https://www.rheumatology.org/Learning-Center/Apps)

ACR Quality Measurement resources (https://www.rheumatology.org/Practice-Quality/Clinical-Support/Quality-Measurement)

The Institute for Healthcare Improvement Web site (www.IHI.org)

CMS' Quality Payment Program Web site (www.qpp.cms.gov)

Rheumatology Informatics System for Effectiveness (RISE) (https://www.rheumatology.org/Practice-Quality/RISE-Registry)

CLINICS CARE POINTS

- Quality measures help improve care by directing quality improvement activities, incentivizing best practices, and assisting patients in selecting health care providers.
- The different types of quality measures have distinct but important roles in improving health care.

DISCLOSURE

Dr. Makris was a VA HSR&D Career Development Awardee at the Dallas VA (CDA 14-425). The views expressed in this article are those of the author(s) and do not necessarily represent the views of the Department of Veterans Affairs.

REFERENCES

1. Berwick DM, Nolan TW, Whittington J. The triple aim: care, health, and cost. Health Aff (Millwood) 2008;27(3):759–69.
2. Bodenheimer T, Sinsky C. From triple to quadruple aim: care of the patient requires care of the provider. Ann Fam Med 2014;12(6):573–6.
3. Nundy S, Cooper LA, Mate KS. The quintuple aim for health care improvement: a new imperative to advance health equity. JAMA 2022;327(6):521.
4. Crossing the quality chasm: a new health system for the 21st century. National Academies Press; 2001. p. 10027. https://doi.org/10.17226/10027.
5. McGlynn EA, Asch SM, Adams J, et al. The Quality of Health Care Delivered to Adults in the United States. N Engl J Med 2003;348(26):2635–45.
6. Gianfrancesco MA, Leykina LA, Izadi Z, et al. Association of Race and Ethnicity With COVID-19 Outcomes in Rheumatic Disease: Data From the COVID-19 Global Rheumatology Alliance Physician Registry. Arthritis Rheumatol Hoboken NJ 2021;73(3):374–80.
7. MacLean CH, Louie R, Leake B, et al. Quality of care for patients with rheumatoid arthritis. JAMA 2000;284(8):984–92.
8. Lim SS, Helmick CG, Bao G, et al. Racial Disparities in Mortality Associated with Systemic Lupus Erythematosus - Fulton and DeKalb Counties, Georgia, 2002-2016. MMWR Morb Mortal Wkly Rep 2019;68(18):419–22.
9. Barton JL, Trupin L, Schillinger D, et al. Racial and ethnic disparities in disease activity and function among persons with rheumatoid arthritis from university-affiliated clinics. Arthritis Care Res 2011;63(9):1238–46.
10. Singh JA, Hodges JS, Toscano JP, et al. Quality of care for gout in the US needs improvement. Arthritis Rheum 2007;57(5):822–9.
11. Ganz DA, Chang JT, Roth CP, et al. Quality of osteoarthritis care for community-dwelling older adults. Arthritis Rheum 2006;55(2):241–7.
12. Curtis JR, Adachi JD, Saag KG. Bridging the osteoporosis quality chasm. J Bone Miner Res Off J Am Soc Bone Miner Res 2009;24(1):3–7.
13. Dooley MA, Hogan S, Jennette C, et al. Cyclophosphamide therapy for lupus nephritis: poor renal survival in black Americans. Glomerular Disease Collaborative Network. Kidney Int 1997;51(4):1188–95.
14. Grigor C, Capell H, Stirling A, et al. Effect of a treatment strategy of tight control for rheumatoid arthritis (the TICORA study): a single-blind randomised controlled trial. Lancet Lond Engl 2004;364(9430):263–9.
15. Verstappen SMM, Jacobs JWG, van der Veen MJ, et al. Intensive treatment with methotrexate in early rheumatoid arthritis: aiming for remission. Computer

Assisted Management in Early Rheumatoid Arthritis (CAMERA, an open-label strategy trial). Ann Rheum Dis 2007;66(11):1443–9.

16. Perez-Ruiz F, Moreno-Lledó A, Urionagüena I, et al. Treat to target in gout. Rheumatol Oxf Engl 2018;57(suppl_1):i20–6.

17. Kim WJ, Song JS, Choi ST. The role of a "treat-to-target" approach in the long-term renal outcomes of patients with gout. J Clin Med 2019;8(7):E1067.

18. Fessler BJ, Alarcón GS, McGwin G, et al. Systemic lupus erythematosus in three ethnic groups: XVI. Association of hydroxychloroquine use with reduced risk of damage accrual. Arthritis Rheum 2005;52(5):1473–80.

19. Brinkmann GH, Norvang V, Norli ES, et al. Treat to target strategy in early rheumatoid arthritis versus routine care - a comparative clinical practice study. Semin Arthritis Rheum 2019;48(5):808–14.

20. Fransen J, Laan RFJM, Van Der Laar MaFJ, et al. Influence of guideline adherence on outcome in a randomised controlled trial on the efficacy of methotrexate with folate supplementation in rheumatoid arthritis. Ann Rheum Dis 2004;63(10):1222–6.

21. Jamal S, Alibhai SMH, Badley EM, et al. Time to treatment for new patients with rheumatoid arthritis in a major metropolitan city. J Rheumatol 2011;38(7):1282–8.

22. MacLean CH, Saag KG, Solomon DH, et al. Measuring quality in arthritis care: methods for developing the Arthritis Foundation's quality indicator set. Arthritis Rheum 2004;51(2):193–202.

23. Chassin MR, Loeb JM, Schmaltz SP, et al. Accountability measures–using measurement to promote quality improvement. N Engl J Med 2010;363(7):683–8.

24. Kiefe CI, Allison JJ, Williams OD, et al. Improving quality improvement using achievable benchmarks for physician feedback. A randomized controlled trial. Am J Ophthalmol 2001;132(5):808.

25. Guidelines and Quality Measures | CDC. 2020. Available at: https://www.cdc.gov/nchhstp/highqualitycare/guidelines-and-quality-measures.html. Accessed December 25, 2021.

26. Donabedian A. Evaluating the quality of medical care. 1966. Milbank Q 2005;83(4):691–729.

27. Donabedian A. The quality of care: how can it be assessed? JAMA 1988;260(12):1743–8.

28. Yazdany J, MacLean CH. Quality of care in the rheumatic diseases: current status and future directions. Curr Opin Rheumatol 2008;20(2):159–66.

29. About Us – OMERACT. Available at: https://omeract.org/about-us/. Accessed February 21, 2022.

30. Barber CEH, Zell J, Yazdany J, et al. American College of Rheumatology Recommended Patient-Reported Functional Status Assessment Measures in Rheumatoid Arthritis. Arthritis Care Res 2019;71(12):1531–9.

31. Quality Measures | CMS. Available at: https://www.cms.gov/Medicare/Quality-Initiatives-Patient-Assessment-Instruments/QualityMeasures. Accessed February 21, 2022.

32. FitzGerald JD, Mikuls TR, Neogi T, et al. Development of the American College of Rheumatology Electronic Clinical Quality Measures for Gout. Arthritis Care Res 2018;70(5):659–71.

33. Clinical Practice Guidelines. Available at: https://www.rheumatology.org/Practice-Quality/Clinical-Support/Clinical-Practice-Guidelines. Accessed February 21, 2022.

34. Institute of Medicine (US). Committee on standards for developing trustworthy clinical practice guidelines. In: Graham R, Mancher M, Miller Wolman D, et al,

editors. Clinical practice guidelines we can trust. National Academies Press (US); 2011. Available at: http://www.ncbi.nlm.nih.gov/books/NBK209539/. Accessed February 21, 2022.

35. Brook RH. The RAND/UCLA appropriateness method. In: Methodology perspectives, AHCPR pub No 95-009. Public health service. U.S. Department of Health and Human Services; 1994. p. 59–70.

36. Goodman SM, Sculco PK. How appropriate are appropriate-use criteria? J Rheumatol 2019;46(9):1064–6.

37. Brook RH, Chassin MR, Fink A, et al. A method for the detailed assessment of the appropriateness of medical technologies. Int J Technol Assess Health Care 1986; 2(1):53–63.

38. Yazdany J, Myslinski R, Miller A, et al. Methods for Developing the American College of Rheumatology's Electronic Clinical Quality Measures: ACR Electronic Clinical Quality Measures. Arthritis Care Res 2016;68(10):1402–9.

39. NQF: NQF's Work in Quality measurement. Available at: https://www.qualityforum. org/about_nqf/work_in_quality_measurement/. Accessed February 21, 2022.

40. HIT and Data Certification. NCQA. Available at: https://www.ncqa.org/programs/ data-and-information-technology/hit-and-data-certification/. Accessed February 21, 2022.

41. NQF: ABCs of Measurement. Available at: https://www.qualityforum.org/ Measuring_Performance/ABCs_of_Measurement.aspx. Accessed February 21, 2022.

42. AHRQ Quality Indicator Tools for Data Analytics. Available at: https://www.ahrq. gov/data/qualityindicators/index.html. Accessed February 21, 2022.

43. Saag KG, Yazdany J, Alexander C, et al. Defining quality of care in rheumatology: The American College of Rheumatology white paper on quality measurement: ACR White Paper on Quality Measurement. Arthritis Care Res 2011;63(1):2–9.

44. Desai SP, Yazdany J. Quality measurement and improvement in rheumatology: rheumatoid arthritis as a case study. Arthritis Rheum 2011;63(12):3649–60.

45. Yazdany J, Robbins M, Schmajuk G, et al. Development of the American College of Rheumatology's Rheumatoid Arthritis Electronic Clinical Quality Measures. Arthritis Care Res 2016;68(11):1579–90.

46. Mant J. Process versus outcome indicators in the assessment of quality of health care. Int J Qual Health Care J Int Soc Qual Health Care 2001;13(6):475–80.

47. Glance LG, Joynt Maddox K, Johnson K, et al. National quality forum guidelines for evaluating the scientific acceptability of risk-adjusted clinical outcome measures: a report from the national quality forum scientific methods panel. Ann Surg 2020;271(6):1048–55.

48. Suter LG, Barber CE, Herrin J, et al. American College of Rheumatology White Paper on Performance Outcome Measures in Rheumatology. Arthritis Care Res 2016;68(10):1390–401.

49. Yazdany J, Bansback N, Clowse M, et al. Rheumatology Informatics System for Effectiveness: A National Informatics-Enabled Registry for Quality Improvement: using RISE Registry to Improve Quality of Care. Arthritis Care Res 2016;68(12): 1866–73.

50. RISE Registry. Available at: https://www.rheumatology.org/Practice-Quality/RISE-Registry. Accessed February 21, 2022.

51. Izadi Z, Schmajuk G, Gianfrancesco M, et al. Significant gains in rheumatoid arthritis quality measures among RISE Registry Practices. Arthritis Care Res 2022;74(2):219–28.

52. Schmajuk G, Li J, Evans M, et al. RISE registry reveals potential gaps in medication safety for new users of biologics and targeted synthetic DMARDs. Semin Arthritis Rheum 2020;50(6):1542–8.
53. Find Healthcare Providers: Compare Care Near You | Medicare. Available at: https://www.medicare.gov/care-compare/. Accessed February 21, 2022.
54. Ovretveit J, Keller C, Hvitfeldt Forsberg H, et al. Continuous innovation: developing and using a clinical database with new technology for patient-centred care–the case of the Swedish quality register for arthritis. Int J Qual Health Care J Int Soc Qual Health Care 2013;25(2):118–24.
55. QPP Overview - QPP. Available at: https://qpp.cms.gov/about/qpp-overview. Accessed February 21, 2022.
56. Department of Health and Human Services Centers for Medicare & Medicaid Services 42 CFR Parts 403, 405, 410, 411, 414, 415, 423, 424, and 425 (2021). Available at: https://www.govinfo.gov/content/pkg/FR-2021-11-19/pdf/2021-23972. pdf. Accessed March 15, 2022.
57. Austin JM, McGlynn EA, Pronovost PJ. Fostering transparency in outcomes, quality, safety, and costs. JAMA 2016;316(16):1661.
58. Berwick DM. Era 3 for Medicine and Health Care. JAMA 2016;315(13):1329.
59. CAHPS for MIPS Survey | CMS. Available at: https://www.cms.gov/Research-Statistics-Data-and-Systems/Research/CAHPS/MIPS. Accessed February 21, 2022.
60. Bermas BL. The emperor has no ganey. Ann Intern Med 2022. https://doi.org/10. 7326/M21-4075.
61. FitzGerald JD, Dalbeth N, Mikuls T, et al. American College of Rheumatology Guideline for the Management of Gout. Arthritis Care Res 2020;72(6):744–60.

Recommendations for Systemic Lupus Erythematosus

Balancing Evidence and Eminence to Facilitate the Medical Care of a Complex Disease

George Bertsias, MD, PhD[a,b]

KEYWORDS

- Lupus nephritis • Glucocorticoids • Consensus • Randomized clinical trials

KEY POINTS

- High-quality, evidence- and eminence-based recommendations exist for systemic lupus erythematosus (SLE) including neuropsychiatric and renal lupus.
- Despite increasing number of controlled and randomized data, there is low evidence base to guide a number of diagnostic, therapeutic, and monitoring decisions in SLE.
- The choice and dosage of treatments may be influenced by regional and ethnic characteristics, which should be considered in the development of SLE recommendations.

INTRODUCTION

Owing to its systemic nature with multiple organs potentially being affected concurrently or sequentially and at varying degrees of severity, the management of systemic lupus erythematosus (SLE) poses significant challenges.[1] Patients with SLE are managed with various compounds including nonsteroid anti-inflammatory drugs, glucocorticoids, synthetic disease-modifying antirheumatic, immunosuppressive and cytotoxic drugs, and more recently, biological agents. During the previous decades, most therapeutic decisions were not supported by high-quality evidence as a consequence of the low disease prevalence and the scantness of randomized data. In this respect, patients with lupus were (and to large extent, are still) seen at referral centers or specialized clinics with interest and expertise in lupus. As a matter of fact, some of these centers have introduced empirical treatment algorithms comprising specific immunosuppressive agents and dosages depending on the clinical presentation.[2,3]

[a] Rheumatology and Clinical Immunology, University of Crete Medical School, Heraklion 71008, Greece; [b] Institute of Molecular Biology and Biotechnology, Foundation for Research and Technology – Hellas (FORTH), Heraklion, Greece
E-mail address: gbertsias@uoc.gr

Rheum Dis Clin N Am 48 (2022) 617–636
https://doi.org/10.1016/j.rdc.2022.05.001
0889-857X/22/© 2022 Elsevier Inc. All rights reserved.

To further complicate matters, multiple medical disciplines (eg, general practitioners, nephrologists, hematologists) can be involved in the diagnosis and treatment of SLE, with often different preferences and practices regarding the selection of immunosuppressive agent, dosage of glucocorticoids, monitoring of treatment response, and assessment of disease outcomes.[4] In an attempt to standardize the medical care—even, the terminology used—and assist the treating physicians, a number of *ad hoc* committees and study groups formed by national and international organizations including the American College of Rheumatology (ACR) and the European Alliance of Associations for Rheumatology (EULAR) have produced over the years multiple sets of recommendations on the management of SLE based on critical analysis of the available evidence and consensus between experts. In this review, I provide a quick reference to these recommendations highlighting a few notable differences and how low-level evidence has been addressed. Additional challenges that are particularly relevant to the disease are also discussed, followed by a perspective view on the future of SLE recommendations.

AN OVERVIEW OF THE RECOMMENDATIONS FOR THE MANAGEMENT OF SYSTEMIC LUPUS ERYTHEMATOSUS

In 1999, the ACR published the first set of guidelines focusing on diagnostic, treatment, and monitoring aspects of SLE and with a target audience of primary care physicians.[5] This article represented a concise—yet comprehensive—overview of multiple disease aspects and it actually underscored a number of concepts that are still considered important and clinically relevant such as early diagnosis and referral, assessment of disease severity, definition of mild lupus, indications for kidney biopsy, the importance for a strategic management plan, the choice of treatments, and monitoring disease activity and potential drug-related toxicity. A few years later, in 2008, a study group used the EULAR standardized operating procedures to produce recommendations for the management of SLE divided into nonmajor and major organ (neuropsychiatric, nephritis) diseases.[6] Other covered topics were the antiphospholipid syndrome (APS), pregnancy, comorbidities, and prognosis of lupus. Despite the fact that several statements were supported by a low evidence base, this article was deemed successful in bringing together several European experts and reconciling their views on challenging topics, such as the indications for immunosuppressive treatment of neuropsychiatric disease, the use of cyclophosphamide versus mycophenolate as induction treatment in lupus nephritis, and the intensity of anticoagulation treatment in APS.[6] Other statements, however, were criticized for being generic and not providing specific guidance to the practicing physicians (eg, risk stratification, glucocorticoids use, and tapering).

In the following years, the community witnessed an increasing number of well conducted, long-term observational and controlled studies, including successful randomized-controlled trials (RCTs) leading to the approval of the first biological agent (belimumab) in 2011.[7,8] This accrual of evidence enabled an in-depth approach to additional clinical aspects such as the optimal use of glucocorticoids,[9,10] the treatment of organ-specific lupus[11] or according to severity stratification, and the indications for initiation of biological agents. This prompted a new series of SLE recommendations starting from the British Society of Rheumatology (BSR)[12,13] and the Latin American Group for the Study of Lupus (GLADEL [Grupo Latino Americano de Estudio del Lupus])–Pan-American League of Associations of Rheumatology (PANLAR)[14,15] in 2018, followed by the updated 2019 EULAR recommendations.[16] In 2021, the Asia-Pacific League of Associations for Rheumatology

(APLAR) SLE special interest group also published their consensus statements on the management in SLE.[17]

KEY DIFFERENCES AMONG THE SYSTEMIC LUPUS ERYTHEMATOSUS RECOMMENDATIONS

Previously, Tunnicliffe and colleagues[18] and Oliveira *and colleagues*[19] have systematically evaluated the methodological quality of each of the general SLE guidelines using the Appraisal of Guidelines for Research and Evaluation II tool. Certain differences in the structure, format, and content of the four aforementioned recommendations are discussed and outlined in **Tables 1** and **2**. All but the BSR recommendations provide overarching principles that generally highlight the need for multidisciplinary and patient-tailored care and he ultimate goals of treatment should include the prevention of organ damage and improvement of survival and health-related quality of life. With the exception of the GLADEL-PANLAR statements that deal only with the treatment of active lupus manifestations, the other recommendations discuss also patient monitoring and the management or prevention of major comorbidities. Owing to the increased burden of infectious complications in SLE patients from the Asia-Pacific region, the APLAR emphasizes infection preventative strategies.[17] Only the BSR guidelines included statements on SLE diagnosis, although both the BSR and the EULAR recommend the use of validated activity instruments (such as the SLE Disease Activity Index [SLEDAI], British Isles Lupus Assessment Group [BILAG]) in disease assessment and patient stratification for treatment selection. Indeed, the BSR was the first to propose different treatment modalities according to SLE activity level (mild, moderate, and severe),[13] a concept that also exists in the 2019 EULAR recommendations.[16]

In terms of specific treatment recommendations (see **Table 2**), a first notable difference pertains to the dose of hydroxychloroquine which should not exceed 6.5 mg/kg/d according to the BSR versus 5 mg/kg/d (actual body weight) and the EULAR and APLAR, whereas the GLADEL provides no recommended dosages for any of the medications. The recommendation for reduced (5 mg/kg) hydroxychloroquine dose was largely based on a single study by Melles *and colleagues*,[20] which was not considered by the BSR. To this end, the corresponding statement is supported by a level of evidence (LoE) 2b with grade of evidence (GoE) C and[16] has triggered debate[21] and the EULAR acknowledges that *"it remains to be confirmed whether a lower [hydroxychloroquine] dose will have comparable clinical effects."*[16]

Another variation between the different sets of guidelines pertains to the initial (starting) recommended dose of glucocorticoids for the management of active/flaring SLE. Thus, the APLAR specifies the dose only for the treatment of active renal (0.6 mg/kg of prednisone equivalent per day) and neuropsychiatric (0.6–1.0 mg/kg per day) disease,[17] whereas the BSR offers specific guidance on the dosage and route of administration (oral, intramuscular, intravenous pulses) according to the degree of SLE activity/severity.[12,13] The EULAR gives a more liberal recommendation that glucocorticoids dose should be tailored to disease severity (no details) and that intravenous pulses of methylprednisolone can be considered especially in the setting of acute organ-threatening disease.[16] Of note, the aforementioned statements by the BSR and the EULAR are supported by low-to-modest non-randomized evidence (LoE/GoE: 2+/C and 3 b/C, respectively) emphasizing the need for additional well designed studies.

All four recommendations have included the use of belimumab for patients with active disease (excluding renal and neurologic lupus) despite conventional therapy. Although the drug efficacy is supported by several RCTs and observational

Table 1
Methodology aspects in published recommendations for the management of systemic lupus erythematosus

	BSR	GLADEL–PANLAR	EULAR	APLAR
Publication year	2018	2018	2019	2021
Scope	Diagnosis, assessment, monitoring, and treatment of non-renal SLE	Treatment of SLE focusing on Latin American population	Assessment, monitoring, and treatment of SLE	Management of SLE in Asia-Pacific region
Target audience	Rheumatologists, other clinicians who care for lupus patients, other allied health professionals	Specialists (not clearly stated)	Rheumatologists, other clinicians who care for lupus patients	Specialists, family physicians, specialty nurses, and other health care professionals
Recommendations development	BSR protocol for guidelines and EULAR standardized operating procedures	Guided by an ad hoc core methods group	EULAR standardized operating procedures	Multiple Delphi rounds
Literature review	Up to 06/2015	Up to 04/2016	Up to 12/2017	Up to 04/2020
Grading of evidence	SIGN	GRADE	CEBM	GRADE
Strength of agreement among experts	Yes (0–10)	Not reported	Yes (0–10)	Yes (0%–100%)
Overarching principles	No	Yes	Yes	Yes
Diagnosis of SLE	Yes	No	No	No
SLE assessment and severity stratification	Yes; instruments (SLEDAI, BILAG); treatment strategies in mild, moderate, and severe SLE	No	Yes; instruments (SLEDAI, PhGA, BILAG)—specific manifestations; treatment strategies in mild, moderate, and severe SLE	Yes (major vs nonmajor organ disease)
Monitoring disease	Yes; details provided on frequency intervals, disease manifestations, serologic tests, drug toxicity, and co-morbidities	No	Yes (use of activity instruments—targets of treatment)	Yes (validated activity instruments; treatment response; drug-related harms; prevention of comorbidities)

Special topics included				
APS	No	Yes	Yes	Yes
Pediatric SLE	No	Childhood-onset lupus nephritis	No	No
Pregnancy in SLE	No separate statements; monitoring is discussed and safety of treatments	No	No	No
Comorbidities	Brief reference	No	Yes (cardiovascular, infections)	Yes (cardiovascular, bone health, emphasis on infections)
Research agenda	Yes	Yes	Yes	No

Abbreviations: ACR, American College of Rheumatology; BILAG, British Isles Lupus Assessment Group; BSR, British Society of Rheumatology; CEBM, Oxford Centre for Evidence-Based Medicine; EULAR, European Alliance of Associations for Rheumatology; GLADEL-PANLAR, Latin American Group for the Study of Lupus (Grupo Latino Americano de Estudio del Lupus)–Pan-American League of Associations of Rheumatology; GRADE, Grading quality of evidence and strength of recommendations; PhGA, Physician Global Assessment; SIGN, Scottish Intercollegiate Guidelines Network; SLE, systemic lupus erythematosus; SLEDAI, SLE Disease Activity Index.

Table 2
Differences in selected topics included in the general systemic lupus erythematosus recommendations

	BSR	GLADEL–PANLAR	EULAR	APLAR
HCQ dose	≤6.5 mg/kg/d	Not reported	≤5 mg/kg/d (actual body weight)	≤5 mg/kg/d (actual body weight)
GC dose	*Mild disease:* topical; or oral prednisolone ≤20 mg/d for 1–2 wk; or i.m. MP 80–120 mg. *Moderate disease:* ≤0.5 mg/d; or i.v. MP ≤250 mg x1–3 d; or i.m. MP 80–120 mg. *Severe disease:* prednisolone ≤0.5 mg/d and/or i.v. MP 500 mg x1–3 d; or prednisolone 0.75–1 mg/kg/d	Not reported	Dose tailored to disease severity (no details) I.v. MP 250–1000 mg/d for 3 d in acute organ-threatening disease	The minimal effective dose of glucocorticoids should be used. Prednisolone 0.6 mg/kg/d (lupus nephritis), 0.6–1.0 mg/kg/d (neuropsychiatric lupus)
Immunosuppressives	MTX (mild, moderate disease); AZA, MMF, CsA (moderate, severe); CY (severe)	Selection according to specific organ involvement	MTX and AZA (mild, moderate disease); CNIs (moderate disease); MMF (moderate, severe disease); CY (severe disease)	MTX, AZA, MMF, CNI (mild, moderate disease; maintenance of severe disease); CY (severe disease)
Indications for belimumab	Refractory moderate disease or severe disease: patients must have positive anti-dsDNA, low complement and an SLEDAI ≥10 despite standard therapy	Refractory musculoskeletal, cutaneous)	Inadequate control (ongoing disease activity or frequent flares) to first-line treatments (typically including combination of HCQ and prednisone with or without immunosuppressive agents), and inability to taper prednisone to maximum 7.5 mg/d	Active SLE manifestations that are refractory to standard therapies (excluding severe disease not included in the trials)

Indications for rituximab	Refractory moderate or severe disease): two or more systems with BILAG B scores, or severe BILAG A activity, or SLEDAI >6, if they have failed two or more immunosuppressive agents (due to inefficacy or intolerance), at least one of which must be MMF or CY; or need for unacceptably high doses of steroids to achieve lower level of disease activity	Diffuse alveolar hemorrhage, neuropsychiatric, refractory hemolytic anemia or thrombocytopenia	Severe renal or extrarenal (mainly hematological, neuropsychiatric) disease refractory to other immunosuppressive agents and/or belimumab, or in patients with contraindications to these drugs	Refractory lupus nephritis and neuropsychiatric disease, or other serious or life-threatening manifestations
Maintenance dosages	Provided for all immunosuppressives; prednisone ≤7.5 mg/d	Not provided	Not provided; prednisone ≤7.5 mg/d	Dose of MMF should be adjusted to body weight
Organ-specific treatment recommendations	No; neuropsychiatric manifestations discussed under severe SLE disease	Yes	Yes	Yes
Treatment target	Ultimate aim to reduce and stop drugs except HCQ eventually when in stable remission	Remission or low-disease activity (overarching principle)	Remission or low-disease activity (validated definitions)	Remission; when remission cannot be achieved, the lowest possible disease activity state should be targeted (validated definitions)

Abbreviations: ACR, American College of Rheumatology; Anti-dsDNA, anti-double strand DNA antibodies; AZA, azathioprine; BILAG, British Isles Lupus Assessment Group; BSR, British Society of Rheumatology; CNI, calcineurin inhibitor; CsA, cyclosporin A; CY, cyclophosphamide; EULAR, European Alliance of Associations for Rheumatology; GLADEL-PANLAR, Latin American Group for the Study of Lupus (Grupo Latino Americano de Estudio del Lupus)–Pan-American League of Associations of Rheumatology; HCQ, hydroxychloroquine; i.m., intramuscular; i.v., intravenous; MMF, mycophenolate mofetil (or equivalent dose of mycophenolic acid); MP, methyl-prednisolone; MTX, methotrexate; SLE, systemic lupus erythematosus; SLEDAI, SLE Disease Activity Index.

studies,[22–25] the community is still struggling to define the subgroups of patients who may benefit the most from belimumab and thus maximize its cost-effectiveness. In this regard and possibly reflecting the different interpretation and views of the expert panels on the drug effectiveness, safety and cost of treatment, the indications for belimumab treatment are different between the four papers. Specifically, the APLAR provides the most generic statement (active SLE manifestations that are refractory to standard therapies excluding severe disease not included in the trials[17]) followed by the EULAR who recommends belimumab for patients with inadequate disease control (ie, persistent disease activity or frequent flares) to first-line treatments typically including combination of hydroxychloroquine and prednisone (with or without immunosuppressive agents) and inability to taper glucocorticoids to 7.5 mg/d or less.[16] The GLADEL recommends the drug in active refractory musculoskeletal and cutaneous disease,[15] probably because of the more robust trial data for these particular manifestations. Finally, the BSR advocates for the use of belimumab only in serologically active (ie, positive anti-double strand DNA antibodies, low complement) patients with high disease activity (Safety of Estrogens in Lupus Erythematosus: National Assessment [SELENA]-SLEDAI score of $\geq$10) because of the larger treatment effect size within this subgroup.[26]

RECOMMENDATIONS FOR LUPUS NEPHRITIS AND IMPORTANT DIFFERENCES

Renal disease represents the most frequent major organ involvement in SLE and is associated with substantial clinical burden and reduced life expectancy.[27] Lupus nephritis is typically diagnosed with kidney biopsy, which is an invasive procedure, its treatment typically requires high-dose glucocorticoids and high-potency immunosuppressive agents, disease monitoring is based on a variety of parameters (eg, serum albumin, glomerular filtration rate, serum electrolytes), and patients can sometimes progress into end-stage kidney disease requiring dialysis or even, kidney transplantation. Based on these distinctive features and the accruing evidence from RCTs specifically designed for patients with active lupus nephritis, the ACR,[28] EULAR jointly with the European Renal Association–European Dialysis and Transplant Association (ERA-EDTA),[29–31] Kidney Disease Improving Global Outcomes (KDIGO),[32] and other societies[33,34] have published specific guidelines for the diagnosis, treatment, and monitoring of lupus nephritis. Focusing on the former three sets of recommendations and despite the fact that these were produced at different periods (the latest versions published in 2012, 2019, and 2021, respectively), they share common characteristics in terms of their format (for instance, the management of proliferative nephritis is presented separately from pure membranous nephritis) and the analyzed evidence base (**Table 3**). Contrary to the ACR and the KDIGO, the joint EULAR/ERA-EDTA initiative comprised a balanced panel of rheumatologists and nephrologists/nephropathologists.

For active proliferative (International Society of Nephrology/Renal Pathology Society [ISN/RPS] class III or IV, with or without coexisting features of class V disease) nephritis, mycophenolate mofetil (or mycophenolic acid) or low-dose intravenous cyclophosphamide (so-called "Euro-lupus") is universally recommended as initial treatment, both agents administered in combination with high-dose glucocorticoids. The standard (high dose) intravenous cyclophosphamide regimen is also included as first-line option in the 2012 ACR recommendations,[28] although it is reserved for the most severe cases (such as with rapidly deteriorating renal function or with crescents in kidney histology) in the 2019 EULAR/ERA-EDTA[30] and the 2021 KDIGO recommendations.[32] This variation might be due to the fact that by 2012 the ACR, representing rheumatologists and rheumatology health professionals predominantly

Table 3
Lupus nephritis recommendations

	ACR 2012	EULAR/ERA-EDTA 2019	KDIGO 2021
Indications for diagnostic kidney biopsy	Increasing serum creatinine; proteinuria ≥1.0 g/24h; proteinuria ≥0.5 g/24h plus hematuria or cellular casts	Any sign of kidney involvement (glomerular hematuria and/or cellular casts, proteinuria >0.5 g/24h (or spot urine protein-to-creatine ratio >500 mg/g), unexplained decrease in GFR)	Abnormal proteinuria (dipstick protein ≥2+ or +1 with low specific gravity), or spot protein-to-creatine ratio >500 mg/g, with/without urine sediment positive for dysmorphic red blood cells, red blood cell or white blood cell casts, further confirmed with 24h protein collection ≥500 mg/d; decreasing GFR

Active proliferative (ISN Class III/IV) LN

	ACR 2012	EULAR/ERA-EDTA 2019	KDIGO 2021
Initial (induction) treatment	MMF (3 g/d [2 g/d in Asians] x6 months—preferred in African-American and Hispanics), or low-dose i.v. CY (0.5 g q2 weeks x6 doses; preferred in European whites), or high-dose i.v. CY (0.5–1 g/m² per month x6) *PLUS* i.v. MP pulses (0.5–1 g x3 days), then oral prednisone 0.5–1 mg/kg/d (1 mg/kg if crescents)	MMF (target dose: 2–3 g/d) or low-dose i.v. CY (500 mg q2 weeks x6 doses) *PLUS* i.v. MP pulses (500–2500 mg, depending on disease severity), followed by oral prednisone (0.3–0.5 mg/kg/d) for up to 4 wk, tapered to ≤7.5 mg/d by 3–6 mo	MMF (2–3 g/d) or i.v. CY (500 mg q2 weeks x6 doses) *PLUS* i.v. MP pulses (0.25–0.5 g × 3 days), then oral prednisone 0.6–1 mg/kg/d; taper to ≤7.5 mg/d by end of 3 mo (* the options of belimumab or CNIs + MMF are discussed but not evaluated)
Severe nephritis	Crescentic: i.v. MP pulses, then oral prednisone 1 mg/kg/d	Combination of MMF (target dose: 1–2 g/d) with CNI (especially TAC) is an alternative, particularly in cases with nephrotic-range proteinuria. Patients at high risk for kidney failure (reduced GFR, histologic presence of crescents or fibrinoid necrosis or severe interstitial inflammation): consider also high-dose i.v. CY (0.5–0.75 g/m² monthly for 6 mo)	Thrombotic microangiopathy (high thrombotic thrombocytopenic purpura risk score): plasma exchange and high-dose glucocorticoids. Standard-dose CY for patients in whom kidney function is rapidly deteriorating and whose biopsy shows severe activity (eg, capillary necrosis, an abundance of crescents).

(continued on next page)

Table 3
(continued)

	ACR 2012	EULAR/ERA-EDTA 2019	KDIGO 2021
Subsequent (maintenance) treatment	MMF or AZA	If improvement after initial treatment is achieved, consider either MMF (1–2 g/d; especially used as initial treatment) or AZA (2 mg/kg/d; preferred if pregnancy is contemplated), in combination with low-dose prednisone (2.5–5 mg/d) when needed to control disease activity	MMF 1–2 g; Selected cases: AZA 1.5–2 mg/d; Lack tolerance: TAC or CsA or mizoribine
Assessment of response to treatment	Physician adjudication; 6 mo (unless there is clear worsening at 3 mo)	Treatment aims for optimization (preservation or improvement) of kidney function, accompanied by a reduction in proteinuria of at least 25% by 3 mo, 50% by 6 mo, and a proteinuria target below 500–700 mg/g by 12 mo (*complete clinical response*) Patients with nephrotic-range proteinuria may require an additional 6–12 mo to reach complete clinical response; in such cases, prompt switches of therapy are not necessary if proteinuria is improving	*Complete renal response*: reduction in proteinuria <0.5 g/g (through 24-h urine collection); stabilization or improvement in kidney function ($\pm$15% of baseline); within the 6–12 mo (but it could take >12 mo) *Partial renal response*: reduction by at least 50% and to <3 g/g; stabilization; within 6–12 mo *No response*: failure to achieve renal response within 6–12 mo of starting therapy
Active membranous (ISN Class V) LN	*Nephrotic-range proteinuria*: prednisone (0.5 mg/kg/d) *PLUS* MMF (2–3 g/d)	MMF (2–3 g/d) *PLUS* pulse i.v. MP (500–2500 mg, depending on disease severity) followed by oral prednisone (20 mg/d, tapered to ≤5 mg/d by 3 mo) Alternative options include i.v. CY, or CNIs (especially TAC) in monotherapy or in combination with MMF, particularly in patients with nephrotic-range proteinuria	*Nephrotic syndrome*: glucocorticoids *PLUS* MMF or CY or CNIs or RTX or AZA *Low-level proteinuria*: immunosuppressive treatment guided by extra-renal activity

Subsequent (maintenance) treatment	As in proliferative LN	As in proliferative LN	As in proliferative LN
Treatment withdrawal	—	Gradual withdrawal of treatment (glucocorticoids first, then immunosuppressive drugs) can be attempted after at least 3–5 y therapy in complete clinical response	The total duration of initial plus maintenance immunosuppression for proliferative LN should not be < 36 mo.
Refractory disease	Switch MMF to CYC *PLUS* Pulses i.v. MP; or RTX, CNIs	Treatment may be switched to one of the alternative initial therapies mentioned above, or to RTX	RTX, or combined MMF plus CNI, or extended course i.v. CY pulses
Other topics covered	Adjunct treatment APS nephropathy Pregnancy Monitoring activity of LN	Adjunct treatment APS nephropathy Pregnancy Monitoring activity of LN Repeat kidney biopsy ESRD—transplantation Pediatric LN	

Abbreviations: ACR, American College of Rheumatology; APS, antiphospholipid syndrome; AZA, azathioprine; CNI, calcineurin inhibitors; CsA, cyclosporine A; CY, cyclophosphamide; ESRD, end-stage renal disease; EULAR/ERA-EDTA, European Alliance of Associations for Rheumatology–European Renal Association–European Dialysis and Transplant Association; GFR, glomerular filtration rate; i.v, intravenous; KDIGO, Kidney Disease Improving Global Outcomes; LN, lupus nephritis; MMF, mycophenolate mofetil (or equivalent dose of mycophenolic acid); RTX, rituximab; TAC, tacrolimus.

from America, had limited available evidence for the effectiveness of the low-dose cyclophosphamide regimen in non-whites.

Another notable difference pertains to the dosage of glucocorticoids. Although pulses of intravenous methylprednisolone (range 0.25–1 g × 3 days) are suggested by all three panels, the EULAR/ERA-EDTA proposes a lower starting dose of oral prednisone (0.3–0.5 mg/kg/d) compared with the ACR and KDIGO (0.5–1 mg/kg/d). This recommendation by the EULAR/ERA-EDTA has a LoE/GoE 2 b/C, which is the result of evidence from the MyLupus controlled study[35] and recent trials (eg, with voclosporin[36]) demonstrating satisfactory renal response rates when pulses of intravenous methylprednisolone are followed by ≤ 0.5 mg/kg/d of prednisone, but likely reflects also the paradigm shift in SLE care by rheumatologists who aim at minimizing exposure to glucocorticoids to avoid organ damage accrual.[1,37] Of note, although the KDIGO included in the systematic literature review the successful trials of voclosporin (in combination with mycophenolate)[36] and belimumab (in combination with low-dose cyclophosphamide or mycophenolate),[38] this new evidence was not appraised and was not graded for quality.

For pure membranous (class V) lupus nephritis, all three guidelines[28,30,32] advocate for immunosuppressants in case of nephrotic-range proteinuria; based on expert opinion, the EULAR/ERA-EDTA extends this recommendation to patients with persistent proteinuria greater than 1 g/24 hours despite the optimal use of renin–angiotensin–aldosterone system blockers for at least 3 months.[30] Furthermore, there are variations in the recommended agents and dosing regimens. Thus, the ACR includes mycophenolate in combination with oral prednisone 0.5 mg/kg/d, although additional options are discussed in this article.[28] The EULAR/ERA-EDTA also recommend mycophenolate in combination with intravenous methylprednisolone pulses followed by moderate-dose oral glucocorticoids (prednisone 20 mg/d), with alternative options including intravenous cyclophosphamide and calcineurin inhibitors (as monotherapy or in combination for mycophenolate).[30] The preference for mycophenolate over other drugs is based on the more favorable toxicity profile, extrapolated also from the treatment of proliferative nephritis, rather than evidence for superior efficacy. Interestingly, and owing to the lack of robust comparative data, the KDIGO offers no specific guidance over the selection of the immunosuppressive agent and even includes azathioprine and rituximab as first-line options.[32] Tight control of hypertension and dyslipidemia is emphasized by both the ACR[28] and the EULAR/ERA-EDTA,[30] the latter also recommending prophylactic anticoagulation in cases of nephrotic syndrome with serum albumin less than 20 g/L.

The ACR recommends that renal response is ascertained by the treating physician at 6 months after treatment initiation unless there is clear worsening at 3 months.[28] Similar to the 2012 EULAR/ERA-EDTA recommendations,[29] the KDIGO advocates for at least *partial* renal response (reduction in proteinuria by ≥ 50% and to <3 g/g, with stabilization of the glomerular filtration rate) with in the first 6 to 12 months.[32] Complete response (proteinuria <0.5 g/g) should be achieved within 6 to 12 but it could take more than 12 months. Of note, the 2019 EULAR/ERA-EDTA introduce time-defined (ie, at 3, 6 and 12 months) response criteria which are mainly derived from post hoc analysis of trial data[31,39] (LoE: 2a-b, GoE: B-D) and align with the prevailing concept of treating-to-target in SLE.[40] Still, another statement indicates that patients with nephrotic-range proteinuria may require additional time to reach the aforementioned targets.

RECOMMENDATIONS FOR OTHER ASPECTS IN THE MANAGEMENT OF SYSTEMIC LUPUS ERYTHEMATOSUS PATIENTS

SLE patients often present with a diversity of manifestations from the neuropsychiatric domain, which pose significant diagnostic and therapeutic challenges as only about one-third of these cases are directly related to the underlying disease, their pathogenesis can be inflammatory, thrombotic, or mixed, and therefore, optimal treatment may differ accordingly.[41,42] In 2010, a EULAR task force comprising rheumatologists, neurologists, and neuroradiologists analyzed the existing literature to prepare recommendations for neuropsychiatric SLE.[43] The first part includes statements on the risk stratification, general diagnostic, and therapeutic approach, followed by a second part with detailed discussion on specific neurologic and psychiatric syndromes. Of note, owing to the scantiness of large or controlled studies, several statements were rated with low GoE (ie, D) or they were based on extrapolation from the management of the same syndromes in the general population. Notwithstanding the lack of robust evidence, these recommendations were well received by the community as they provided a useful framework for choosing the appropriate tests (eg, brain magnetic resonance imaging [MRI], cerebrospinal fluid analysis), facilitating the attribution of neuropsychiatric events to SLE or not, and choosing the intensity of immunosuppressive and antithrombotic therapy.[44] In view of new data,[45,46] one of the statements pertaining to the indication for immunosuppressive treatment in lupus-associated cerebrovascular disease was later amended in the 2019 update of the general SLE recommendations to emphasize that immunosuppression *"may be considered in the absence of aPL antibodies and other atherosclerotic risk factors or in recurrent cerebrovascular events,"*[16]

Cutaneous manifestations are often the prevailing disease feature in patients with SLE, thus necessitating more directed treatments. To this end, both the 2018 GLADEL-PANLAR[15] and 2019 EULAR[16] recommendations provide separate statements specifically for the treatment of skin disease with immunosuppressive and biological agents. Of relevance, the EULAR panel included two dermatologists with expertise in cutaneous lupus and the recommended management of refractory skin disease is elaborated with agents such as retinoids and dapsone (both with LoE/GoE 4/C) with thalidomide being discussed in the article as a rescue therapy option.[16] In this context, specific guidelines for the diagnosis and management of cutaneous lupus have been produced by dermatologists (eg, European Dermatology Forum in cooperation with the European Academy of Dermatology and Venereology[47,48]).

Although included to some extent in the abovementioned general recommendations, specific EULAR guidelines exist for other aspects of SLE including disease and patient monitoring in routine practice and observational studies,[49] family planning, assisted reproduction, pregnancy and menopause,[50] and cardiovascular risk management.[51] Similarly, the Canadian Rheumatology Association published in 2018 recommendations on the diagnosis, disease activity, and damage assessment, suggesting the use of a validated disease activity score per visit and annual damage score.[52] They also recommend on specific assessment for the prevention of comorbidities including malignancy and infections. The significance of these guidelines lies in the more comprehensive and granular approach to selected research and clinical questions, aiming to provide as much specific as possible guidance to treating physicians. Finally, large international task forces have addressed additional important topics in SLE such as the goals of treatment toward a treating-to-target approach.[53] In fact, this project paved the way toward a definition of remission[54] in SLE which can be used in the setting of routine care and therapeutic trials. For the sake of completeness, a large panel of French-speaking experts has also generated recommendations on the use of biological agents (belimumab, rituximab, abatacept, tocilizumab) in patients with SLE.[55]

CHALLENGES IN PRODUCING SYSTEMIC LUPUS ERYTHEMATOSUS RECOMMENDATIONS

Despite growing research in SLE, there are a relatively small number of controlled or randomized studies to address the numerous challenges and dilemmas that treating physicians may be confronted with in daily practice. Indeed, low-level evidence can be an important barrier to establishing recommendations that are as much clear and straightforward as possible. Despite these limitations, a decision can be made by the guideline panel to continue working to formulate a statement/recommendation on a topic that is deemed clinically significant. This is exemplified in the case of gluco-corticoids dosage and tapering schemes which vary considerably among the different recommendations and are supported by a GoE of C. The lack of strong evidence inev-itably empowers the eminence-based strategy which is based on the clinical (anec-dotal) experience and personal views of the panelists. Although this process enables capture of the "wisdom" of experienced clinicians, it can sometimes be chal-lenging to reconcile different opinions into a concise statement. From the end-user perspective, physicians should generally feel assured if low evidence statements have a strong level of agreement among experts. To this end, one should bear in mind that the "one size fits all" rule may not always apply in SLE considering the highly heterogeneous nature of the disease. In the same context, the recommendations should leave flexibility to physicians to manage less common or typical clinical scenarios.

Another challenging aspect is the consideration of regional or ethnic differences related to the effectiveness and safety of lupus medications. This was first under-scored by a post hoc analysis of the Aspreva Lupus Management Study trial in lupus nephritis, which revealed that more Black and Hispanic patients responded to myco-phenolate than cyclophosphamide.[56] This observation has resulted in the unanimous recommendation for mycophenolate as first-line therapy for lupus nephritis, whereas there is some variation regarding the use of standard versus low-dose intravenous cyclophosphamide.[17] The recommended dose of mycophenolate also varies between the different guidelines. Although the 2012 EULAR/ERA-EDTA paper suggested a "target" mycophenolate mofetil dose of 3 g/d during the first 6 months,[29] it was appre-ciated initially by the ACR[28] and later, by the EULAR/ERA-EDTA[30] that doses exceeding 2 g/d may not always be tolerated especially by Asian patients. This led to recommending a dose range of mycophenolate mofetil (2–3 g/d or equivalent dose of mycophenolic acid). Moreover, a critical factor to appraise is whether a spe-cific drug has been sufficiently tested in patients with different ethnic backgrounds. For example, initial data on the efficacy of low-dose intravenous cyclophosphamide were exclusively from White patients with active proliferative nephritis,[57,58] although in the following years, the regimen was tested in other ethnicities.[59,60] Likewise, pre-liminary evidence for the use of voclosporin in lupus nephritis originated from studies that included predominantly Asian patients.[61] This caused some initial skepticism for its generalized use, which however, has regressed as the publication of the multiethnic phase III trial results.[36] Some of the considerations, coupled also with variations in the availability or patient access to certain drugs in some regions, are reflected in the GLA-DEL-PANLAR,[15] APLAR,[17] and other[62] recommendations.

As lupus diagnosis and treatment often involves multiple medical disciplines, it is desirable that these are also involved in the production of SLE recommendations by providing their expertise and perspective in selected topics. This approach can help to reduce discrepancies such as for instance, in patterns of glucocorticoids admin-istration, foster closer interaction and eventually, enhance and improve patient care.

The 2012[29] and 2019[30] joint EULAR/ERA-EDTA recommendations represent an example for such collaborative efforts.

RECOMMENDATIONS VERSUS USUAL CARE OF PATIENTS WITH SYSTEMIC LUPUS ERYTHEMATOSUS

Assessing the implementation of guidelines or comparing them against the actual clinical practice is helpful to realize possible limitations or barriers to meet the published standards.[63] A retrospective chart-based evaluation at two tertiary centers of 94 SLE patients who experienced 123 neuropsychiatric events identified certain areas of divergence from the neuropsychiatric SLE (NPSLE) recommendations including the overutilization of brain MRI, the underutilization of the full battery of neuropsychological testing in patients with possible cognitive dysfunction, and the fact that many (52%) patients with cerebrovascular events received both immunosuppressive and antithrombotic therapy because of either coexisting generalized lupus activity or recurrence despite prior antithrombotic treatment.[46] The latter observation together with other supportive evidence led to reconsideration of the indication for immunosuppressive treatment in SLE-associated stroke.[16]

Pearce *and colleagues*[63] conducted a prospective audit in 51 units (both general and dedicated or specialized clinics) in the United Kingdom to evaluate the implementation of the 2018 BSR recommendations. The findings were reflective of the high disease burden as 28.5% had active disease, and glucocorticoids were administered in 49% of the visits. Of note, there was low documented compliance relating to the recommended disease activity assessment, reduction of drug-related toxicity, and prevention of comorbidities and organ damage.[63] Taken together, the implications of these studies are multiple and pertain to revising the feasibility of the recommendations, the identification of areas for quality improvement and actions to cover educational gaps and support decision-making.

SYSTEMIC LUPUS ERYTHEMATOSUS RECOMMENDATIONS: FUTURE PERSPECTIVES

Similar to other rheumatic diseases, research in SLE is rapidly progressing with accruing data from multiple observational studies and RCTs. As a matter of fact, a number of compounds or treatment strategies are currently being investigated in phase II and III trials and hopefully, some of them will yield positive results. Driven by advances in basic and translational research, additional novel targeted treatments and biomarkers for diagnosis, stratification, and prognosis are expected in the near future, which could potentially revolutionize many aspects in SLE care. Therefore, it is expected that SLE recommendations will continue to be revised at regular basis. In addition to the challenges discussed above, the new panels will be required to build on the previously appraised evidence and gained experience to focus on areas of uncertainty with low evidence base and try to upgrade them, improve clarity where needed, and identify emergent topics of relevance to the disease, physicians, and patients. The latter should be placed more centrally to the process including the selection of topics, interpretation of the literature research results, and drafting of the statements and the article.[64] In the future, it is possible that the production of new recommendations will be facilitated by methodologies such as the nominal group technique already used in the development of classification criteria.[65] Even so, the success of the undertaking will rely on the team work and interaction between physicians with clinical and research experience in this complex disease.

CLINICS CARE POINTS

- The treatment of SLE should be tailored to the disease activity and severity adjudicated by physicians and validated clinical instruments.

- Besides disease activity and response to treatment, SLE patients should be monitored regularly for the prevention and optimal management of drug-related harms, especially from glucocorticoids, and comorbidities.

- Biological agents are recommended for SLE patients with persistent disease activity or frequent flares despite conventional therapy (antimalarials, immunosuppressants, glucocorticoids) or inability to taper prednisone dose to less than 7.5 mg/day.

- Initial treatment of active lupus nephritis includes either mycophenolate or low-dose intravenous cyclophosphamide, both in combination with glucocorticoids. High-dose cyclophosphamide should be reserved for aggressive disease.

- Although not appraised by existing recommendations, additional options include the combination of mycophenolate with either belimumab (moderately severe nephritis, extra-renal activity, minimization of glucocorticoids) or calcineurin inhibitors (profound nephrotic syndrome, podocytopathy).

DISCLOSURE

There are no disclosures relevant to this work.

REFERENCES

1. Fanouriakis A, Tziolos N, Bertsias G, Boumpas DT. Update omicronn the diagnosis and management of systemic lupus erythematosus. Ann Rheum Dis 2021;80(1):14–25.
2. Luijten RK, Fritsch-Stork RD, Bijlsma JW, Derksen RH. The use of glucocorticoids in systemic lupus erythematosus. After 60 years still more an art than science. Autoimmun Rev 2013;12(5):617–28.
3. Ruiz-Irastorza G, Bertsias G. Treating systemic lupus erythematosus in the 21st century: new drugs and new perspectives on old drugs. Rheumatology (Oxford) 2020;59(Suppl5):v69–81.
4. Lerang K, Gilboe IM, Gran JT. Differences between rheumatologists and other internists regarding diagnosis and treatment of systemic lupus erythematosus. Rheumatology (Oxford) 2012;51(4):663–9.
5. Guidelines for referral and management of systemic lupus erythematosus in adults. American College of Rheumatology Ad Hoc Committee on Systemic Lupus Erythematosus Guidelines. Arthritis Rheum 1999;42(9):1785–96.
6. Bertsias G, Ioannidis JP, Boletis J, et al. EULAR recommendations for the management of systemic lupus erythematosus. Report of a Task Force of the EULAR Standing Committee for International Clinical Studies Including Therapeutics. Ann Rheum Dis 2008;67(2):195–205.
7. Navarra SV, Guzman RM, Gallacher AE, et al. Efficacy and safety of belimumab in patients with active systemic lupus erythematosus: a randomised, placebo-controlled, phase 3 trial. Lancet 2011;377(9767):721–31.
8. Furie R, Petri M, Zamani O, et al. A phase III, randomized, placebo-controlled study of belimumab, a monoclonal antibody that inhibits B lymphocyte stimulator, in patients with systemic lupus erythematosus. Arthritis Rheum 2011;63(12):3918–30.

9. Ruiz-Arruza I, Ugarte A, Cabezas-Rodriguez I, Medina JA, Moran MA, Ruiz-Irastorza G. Glucocorticoids and irreversible damage in patients with systemic lupus erythematosus. Rheumatology (Oxford) 2014;53(8):1470–6.

10. Al Sawah S, Zhang X, Zhu B, et al. Effect of corticosteroid use by dose on the risk of developing organ damage over time in systemic lupus erythematosus-the Hopkins Lupus Cohort. Lupus Sci Med 2015;2(1):e000066.

11. Sigges J, Biazar C, Landmann A, et al. Therapeutic strategies evaluated by the European Society of Cutaneous Lupus Erythematosus (EUSCLE) Core Set Questionnaire in more than 1000 patients with cutaneous lupus erythematosus. Autoimmun Rev 2013;12(7):694–702.

12. Gordon C, Amissah-Arthur MB, Gayed M, et al. The British Society for Rheumatology guideline for the management of systemic lupus erythematosus in adults. Rheumatology (Oxford) 2018;57(1):e1–45.

13. Gordon C, Amissah-Arthur MB, Gayed M, et al. The British Society for Rheumatology guideline for the management of systemic lupus erythematosus in adults: Executive Summary. Rheumatology (Oxford) 2018;57(1):14–8.

14. Cardiel MH, Soriano ER, Bonfa E, et al. Therapeutic Guidelines for Latin American Lupus Patients: Methodology. J Clin Rheumatol 2018;24(1):41–4.

15. Pons-Estel BA, Bonfa E, Soriano ER, et al. First Latin American clinical practice guidelines for the treatment of systemic lupus erythematosus: Latin American Group for the Study of Lupus (GLADEL, Grupo Latino Americano de Estudio del Lupus)-Pan-American League of Associations of Rheumatology (PANLAR). Ann Rheum Dis 2018;77(11):1549–57.

16. Fanouriakis A, Kostopoulou M, Alunno A, et al. 2019 update of the EULAR recommendations for the management of systemic lupus erythematosus. Ann Rheum Dis 2019;78(6):736–45.

17. Mok CC, Hamijoyo L, Kasitanon N, et al. The Asia-Pacific League of Associations for Rheumatology consensus statements on the management of systemic lupus erythematosus. Lancet Rheumatol 2021;3(7):e517–31.

18. Tunnicliffe DJ, Singh-Grewal D, Kim S, Craig JC, Tong A. Diagnosis, monitoring, and treatment of systemic lupus erythematosus: a systematic review of clinical practice guidelines. Arthritis Care Res (Hoboken) 2015;67(10):1440–52.

19. Oliveira M, Palacios-Fernandez S, Cervera R, Espinosa G. Clinical practice guidelines and recommendations for the management of patients with systemic lupus erythematosus: a critical comparison. Rheumatology (Oxford) 2020; 59(12):3690–9.

20. Melles RB, Marmor MF. The risk of toxic retinopathy in patients on long-term hydroxychloroquine therapy. JAMA Ophthalmol 2014;132(12):1453–60.

21. Costedoat-Chalumeau N, Isenberg D, Petri M. Comment on the 2019 update of the EULAR recommendations for the management of systemic lupus erythematosus by Fanouriakis et al. Ann Rheum Dis 2020;79(8):e90.

22. Depascale R, Gatto M, Zen M, et al. Belimumab: a step forward in the treatment of systemic lupus erythematosus. Expert Opin Biol Ther 2021;21(5):563–73.

23. Fanouriakis A, Adamichou C, Koutsoviti S, et al. Low disease activity-irrespective of serologic status at baseline-associated with reduction of corticosteroid dose and number of flares in patients with systemic lupus erythematosus treated with belimumab: a real-life observational study. Semin Arthritis Rheum 2018; 48(3):467–74.

24. Petrou P. A systematic review of the economic evaluations of belimumab in systemic lupus erythematosus. Value Health Reg Issues 2022;27:32–40.

25. Singh JA, Shah NP, Mudano AS. Belimumab for systemic lupus erythematosus. Cochrane Database Syst Rev 2021;2:CD010668.
26. van Vollenhoven RF, Petri MA, Cervera R, et al. Belimumab in the treatment of systemic lupus erythematosus: high disease activity predictors of response. Ann Rheum Dis 2012;71(8):1343–9.
27. Kostopoulou M, Adamichou C, Bertsias G. An Update on the Diagnosis and Management of Lupus Nephritis. Curr Rheumatol Rep 2020;22(7):30.
28. Hahn BH, McMahon MA, Wilkinson A, et al. American College of Rheumatology guidelines for screening, treatment, and management of lupus nephritis. Arthritis Care Res (Hoboken) 2012;64(6):797–808.
29. Bertsias GK, Tektonidou M, Amoura Z, et al. Joint European League Against Rheumatism and European Renal Association-European Dialysis and Transplant Association (EULAR/ERA-EDTA) recommendations for the management of adult and paediatric lupus nephritis. Ann Rheum Dis 2012;71(11):1771–82.
30. Fanouriakis A, Kostopoulou M, Cheema K, et al. 2019 Update of the Joint European League Against Rheumatism and European Renal Association-European Dialysis and Transplant Association (EULAR/ERA-EDTA) recommendations for the management of lupus nephritis. Ann Rheum Dis 2020;79(6):713–23.
31. Kostopoulou M, Fanouriakis A, Cheema K, et al. Management of lupus nephritis: a systematic literature review informing the 2019 update of the joint EULAR and European Renal Association-European Dialysis and Transplant Association (EULAR/ERA-EDTA) recommendations. RMD Open 2020;6(2):e001263.
32. Kidney Disease: Improving Global Outcomes Glomerular Diseases Work G. KDIGO 2021 Clinical Practice Guideline for the Management of Glomerular Diseases. Kidney Int 2021;100(4S):S1–276. https://doi.org/10.1016/j.kint.2021.05.021.
33. van Tellingen A, Voskuyl AE, Vervloet MG, et al. Dutch guidelines for diagnosis and therapy of proliferative lupus nephritis. Neth J Med 2012;70(4):199–207. https://www.ncbi.nlm.nih.gov/pubmed/22641632.
34. Wilhelmus S, Bajema IM, Bertsias GK, et al. Lupus nephritis management guidelines compared. Nephrol Dial Transplant 2016;31(6):904–13.
35. Zeher M, Doria A, Lan J, et al. Efficacy and safety of enteric-coated mycophenolate sodium in combination with two glucocorticoid regimens for the treatment of active lupus nephritis. Lupus 2011;20(14):1484–93.
36. Rovin BH, Teng YKO, Ginzler EM, et al. Efficacy and safety of voclosporin versus placebo for lupus nephritis (AURORA 1): a double-blind, randomised, multicentre, placebo-controlled, phase 3 trial. Lancet 2021;397(10289):2070–80.
37. Dorner T, Furie R. Novel paradigms in systemic lupus erythematosus. Lancet 2019;393(10188):2344–58.
38. Furie R, Rovin BH, Houssiau F, et al. Two-Year, Randomized, Controlled Trial of Belimumab in Lupus Nephritis. N Engl J Med 2020;383(12):1117–28.
39. Tamirou F, Lauwerys BR, Dall'Era M, et al. A proteinuria cut-off level of 0.7 g/day after 12 months of treatment best predicts long-term renal outcome in lupus nephritis: data from the MAINTAIN Nephritis Trial. Lupus Sci Med 2015;2(1):e000123.
40. Parra Sanchez AR, Voskuyl AE, van Vollenhoven RF. Treat-to-target in systemic lupus erythematosus: advancing towards its implementation. Nat Rev Rheumatol 2022;18(3):146–57.
41. Moore E, Huang MW, Putterman C. Advances in the diagnosis, pathogenesis and treatment of neuropsychiatric systemic lupus erythematosus. Curr Opin Rheumatol 2020;32(2):152–8.

42. Nikolopoulos D, Fanouriakis A, Bertsias G. Treatment of neuropsychiatric systemic lupus erythematosus: clinical challenges and future perspectives. Expert Rev Clin Immunol 2021;17(4):317–30.

43. Bertsias GK, Ioannidis JP, Aringer M, et al. EULAR recommendations for the management of systemic lupus erythematosus with neuropsychiatric manifestations: report of a task force of the EULAR standing committee for clinical affairs. Ann Rheum Dis 2010;69(12):2074–82.

44. Fanouriakis A, Bertsias G, Govoni M. Editorial: lupus and the brain: advances in neuropsychiatric systemic lupus erythematosus. Front Med (Lausanne) 2019; 6:52.

45. Cohen D, Rijnink EC, Nabuurs RJ, et al. Brain histopathology in patients with systemic lupus erythematosus: identification of lesions associated with clinical neuropsychiatric lupus syndromes and the role of complement. Rheumatology (Oxford) 2017;56(1):77–86.

46. Pamfil C, Fanouriakis A, Damian L, et al. EULAR recommendations for neuropsychiatric systemic lupus erythematosus vs usual care: results from two European centres. Rheumatology (Oxford) 2015;54(7):1270–8.

47. Worm M, Zidane M, Eisert L, et al. S2k guideline: Diagnosis and management of cutaneous lupus erythematosus - Part 1: classification, diagnosis, prevention, activity scores. J Dtsch Dermatol Ges 2021;19(8):1236–47.

48. Worm M, Zidane M, Eisert L, et al. S2k guideline: Diagnosis and management of cutaneous lupus erythematosus - Part 2: therapy, risk factors and other special topics. J Dtsch Dermatol Ges 2021;19(9):1371–95.

49. Mosca M, Tani C, Aringer M, et al. European League Against Rheumatism recommendations for monitoring patients with systemic lupus erythematosus in clinical practice and in observational studies. Ann Rheum Dis 2010;69(7):1269–74.

50. Andreoli L, Bertsias GK, Agmon-Levin N, et al. EULAR recommendations for women's health and the management of family planning, assisted reproduction, pregnancy and menopause in patients with systemic lupus erythematosus and/ or antiphospholipid syndrome. Ann Rheum Dis 2017;76(3):476–85.

51. Drosos GC, Vedder D, Houben E, et al. EULAR recommendations for cardiovascular risk management in rheumatic and musculoskeletal diseases, including systemic lupus erythematosus and antiphospholipid syndrome. Ann Rheum Dis 2022. https://doi.org/10.1136/annrheumdis-2021-221733.

52. Keeling SO, Alabdurubalnabi Z, Avina-Zubieta A, et al. Canadian rheumatology association recommendations for the assessment and monitoring of systemic lupus erythematosus. J Rheumatol 2018;45(10):1426–39.

53. van Vollenhoven RF, Mosca M, Bertsias G, et al. Treat-to-target in systemic lupus erythematosus: recommendations from an international task force. Ann Rheum Dis 2014;73(6):958–67.

54. van Vollenhoven R, Voskuyl A, Bertsias G, et al. A framework for remission in SLE: consensus findings from a large international task force on definitions of remission in SLE (DORIS). Ann Rheum Dis 2017;76(3):554–61.

55. Kleinmann JF, Tubach F, Le Guern V, et al. International and multidisciplinary expert recommendations for the use of biologics in systemic lupus erythematosus. Autoimmun Rev 2017;16(6):650–7.

56. Isenberg D, Appel GB, Contreras G, et al. Influence of race/ethnicity on response to lupus nephritis treatment: the ALMS study. Rheumatology (Oxford) 2010;49(1): 128–40.

57. Houssiau FA, Vasconcelos C, D'Cruz D, et al. Immunosuppressive therapy in lupus nephritis: the Euro-Lupus Nephritis Trial, a randomized trial of low-dose

versus high-dose intravenous cyclophosphamide. Arthritis Rheum 2002;46(8): 2121–31.

58. Houssiau FA, Vasconcelos C, D'Cruz D, et al. The 10-year follow-up data of the Euro-Lupus Nephritis Trial comparing low-dose and high-dose intravenous cyclophosphamide. Ann Rheum Dis 2010;69(1):61–4.

59. Wofsy D, Diamond B, Houssiau FA. Crossing the Atlantic: the Euro-Lupus Nephritis regimen in North America. Arthritis Rheumatol 2015;67(5):1144–6.

60. Houssiau FA. Moving East: the Euro-Lupus Nephritis regimen in Asia. Kidney Int 2016;89(1):25–7.

61. Rovin BH, Solomons N, Pendergraft WF 3rd, et al. A randomized, controlled double-blind study comparing the efficacy and safety of dose-ranging voclosporin with placebo in achieving remission in patients with active lupus nephritis. Kidney Int 2019;95(1):219–31.

62. Klumb EM, Scheinberg M, Souza VA, et al. The landscape of systemic lupus erythematosus in Brazil: an expert panel review and recommendations. Lupus 2021;30(10):1684–95.

63. Pearce FA, Rutter M, Sandhu R, et al. BSR guideline on the management of adults with systemic lupus erythematosus (SLE) 2018: baseline multi-centre audit in the UK. Rheumatology (Oxford) 2021;60(3):1480–90.

64. Schneider M. Guidelines for the management of systemic lupus erythematosus: great synthesis of evidence and eminence with limited focus on patient's needs. Rheumatology (Oxford) 2018;57(1):12–3.

65. Johnson SR, Khanna D, Daikh D, et al. Use of consensus methodology to determine candidate items for systemic lupus erythematosus classification criteria. J Rheumatol 2019;46(7):721–6.

Osteoarthritis Treatment Guidelines from Six Professional Societies
Similarities and Differences

Chris Overton, MD[a], Amanda E. Nelson, MD, MSCR[a],
Tuhina Neogi, MD, PhD[b],*

KEYWORDS

- Osteoarthritis • Treatment guidelines • GRADE

KEY POINTS

- Contemporary treatment guidelines for osteoarthritis (OA) published by various professional societies in the past 5 years have used Grading of Recommendations, Assessment, Development and Evaluations (GRADE) methodology, making their approaches more comparable than in the past.
- Each of the recent OA guidelines generally had similar recommendations regarding education, self-management, and physical approaches, as well as recommending oral and topical NSAIDs as the primary pharmacologic approaches.
- There is a paucity of recommended pharmacologic therapies, highlighting a major unmet need in OA management.

INTRODUCTION

Osteoarthritis (OA) affects approximately 500 million people worldwide,[1] and contributes substantially to years lived with disability worldwide.[2] Furthermore, in the United States, OA is the third leading hospital discharge diagnosis after childbirth-related (#1) and sepsis-related (#2) hospitalizations due to the large volume of joint replacements performed annually,[3] highlighting the substantial public health impact of this disease. Despite its prevalence and burden, there are no approved pharmacologic agents to

[a] Division of Rheumatology, Allergy, and Immunology, Thurston Arthritis Research Center, University of North Carolina at Chapel Hill, 3300 Doc J. Thurston Bldg, CB#7280, Chapel Hill, NC 27599, USA; [b] Boston University School of Medicine, 650 Albany Street, Rheumatology, Suite X200, Boston, MA 02118, USA
* Corresponding author.
E-mail address: tneogi@bu.edu
Twitter: @Tuhina_Neogi (T.N.)

Rheum Dis Clin N Am 48 (2022) 637–657
https://doi.org/10.1016/j.rdc.2022.03.009
0889-857X/22/© 2022 Elsevier Inc. All rights reserved.

date that effectively halt disease progression; thus management largely focuses on symptoms.

Numerous treatment guidelines exist for OA from various professional societies across the world. Whereas different methodologies have historically been used to develop treatment guidelines, formal guideline methodology to develop evidence-based guidelines have been generally adopted by professional societies, as advocated by the Institute of Medicine (IOM),[4] and reviewed elsewhere in this issue (see Sindhu R Johnson and colleagues' article, "How the American College of Rheumatology Develops Guidelines," in this issue). To facilitate the translation and implementation of guidelines into practice, we endeavored to evaluate and summarize the most recent treatment guidelines published in the past 5 years, and to examine similarities and differences among them.

METHODS

We performed a literature search to identify OA guidelines published/updated within the past 5 years (search conducted in November, 2021) from major societies. We did not consider surgical management guidelines and did not include articles evaluating single interventions, a single aspect of OA care, diagnosis of OA, or unspecified site of OA in recommendations made, or editorial pieces. Guidelines were selected by 2 expert rheumatologist/epidemiologists (TN and AN); data extraction was performed by TN, AN, and a senior rheumatology fellow (CO). A data extraction form (Excel spreadsheet) was reviewed and edited by all authors. Extracted data included: publication year, country, specialties involved, whether a systematic review was performed, the target users, and whether competing interests were discussed. Each author extracted recommendations from 2 guidelines into a shared document, and the strength of recommendation was recorded. All authors reviewed the extraction tables for accuracy and completeness.

To ease the interpretation of the recommendations, the authors independently reviewed the data extraction tables for all guidelines and converted each guideline's recommendations to a uniform standard of strongly or conditionally recommended for or against, and indicated whereby the intervention was not discussed or no recommendations were made despite consideration.

RESULTS

We identified and selected the following 6 guidelines for OA management, which collectively addressed the management of hand, knee, hip, and polyarticular OA (listed in alphabetical order of the professional society sponsoring the guideline):

- American Academy of Orthopedic Surgeons (AAOS) Management of Osteoarthritis of the Knee (nonarthroplasty) Evidence-Based Clinical Practice Guideline
- American College of Rheumatology/Arthritis Foundation (ACR/AF) Guideline for the Management of Osteoarthritis of the Hand, Hip, and Knee[5,6]
- An updated algorithm recommendation for the management of knee OA from the European Society for Clinical and Economic Aspects of Osteoporosis, Osteoarthritis, and Musculoskeletal Diseases (ESCEO)[7]
- 2018 update of the European Alliance of Associations for Rheumatology (EULAR) recommendations for the management of hand OA[8]
- Osteoarthritis Research Society International (OARSI) guidelines for the nonsurgical management of knee, hip, and polyarticular OA[9]

- Veterans Affairs and Department of Defense (VA/DOD) Clinical Practice Guideline For The Non-Surgical Management Of Hip & Knee Osteoarthritis (accessed at: https://www.healthquality.va.gov/guidelines/CD/OA/VADoDOACPG.pdf)

Three of the guidelines were from the United States, 2 were from Europe, and one included international input from Canada, Europe, Australia, China, and Japan. Two guidelines also included surgical recommendations (AAOS, EULAR hand), which we will not review here. Most recommendations were directed toward physicians and allied health professionals, and most guidelines had multi-disciplinary input from rheumatologists, general practitioners, orthopedists, and physical therapists; some also included physical medicine & rehabilitation specialists, geriatricians, sports medicine, and public health specialists. GRADE methodology was used in all but one guideline (EULAR hand), and all but one (AAOS) had patient representation.

All guidelines had an explicit statement about conflicts of interest with the exception of the AAOS. However, handling of conflicts of interest varied across the guidelines. For example, in some guidelines, like the ACR/AF, at least 50% of guidelines contributors had to be free of any perceived or real conflicts of interest in line with IOM recommendations, whereas others only required a declaration of any potentially relevant conflicts of interest. The issue of potential conflicts of interest among guideline participants has been scrutinized as they can undermine trust in guideline recommendations if not adequately managed.[10]

Terminology

A major set of management options for OA falls under the umbrella of what has traditionally been labeled as "nonpharmacologic" therapies. However, attention should be paid to terminology used to describe those options to engage patients positively in the shared decision-making process. It is increasingly recognized that semantics matter and that active or participatory language is important for patient engagement.[11] For example, describing a therapy as "non-X" prefix, such as "nonpharmacologic" or "nonsurgical," may inadvertently connote those "non-X" therapeutic options to be less effective or preferred than the therapies named after the prefix. Consensus on appropriate terminology to promote positive and empowering language that supports patient engagement in such modalities has not yet been addressed. In the ACR/AF Guideline, the term "nonpharmacologic" was replaced with descriptive terms such as physical, mind-body, and behavioral modalities. We have opted to use the term Physical and Behavioral Modalities to refer to this category of management options.

Physical and Behavioral Modalities

All guidelines made recommendations regarding physical and behavioral modalities, often considering these as foundational to the management of OA. The recommendations can be generally grouped into the following 4 themes: (1) education and self-management, (2) exercise and weight loss, (3) joint support and assistive devices, (4) alternative and complementary modalities. A summary of the recommendations for the knee is shown in **Table 1**, for the hip in **Table 2**, and for the hand in **Table 3**.

Education and self-management

All guidelines made moderate to strong recommendations for education and self-management as part of OA management. The importance of patient education was addressed, including education about the disease, medication effects and potential side effects, joint protection measures, and exercise goals and approaches. Self-efficacy and self-management programs were consistently strongly recommended

Table 1
Physical & behavior modality recommendations for the management of knee osteoarthritis

	OARSI	VA/DoD	ACR/AF	AAOS	ESCEO
Self-management programs and education	Education Self-mgmt				
Weight Loss (if overweight)					
Exercise		nd			
Low-impact aerobic exercise (aquatic and/or land based)	Land-based Aquatic				nd
Yoga; Range of motion/flexibility	nd	nd	Yoga	nd	nd
Supervised exercise with manual therapy	nd	nd			nd
Balance		nd		nd	nd
Manual therapy alone	nd	nd		nd	nd
Group and home equally effective/individualize	nd	no preference	nd	nd	nd
Consider PT/OT referral	nd		nd	nd	mentioned, but no specific GRADE rec
Mobilization and manipulation		nd	nd	nd	nd
neuromuscular training		nd	nd		nd
Joint support and assistive devices					
Patellar taping		nd		nd	nd
Brace with varus/valgus as indicated		a	tibiofemoral Patellofemoral		nd
Heel wedges (medial or lateral as indicated)		nd		lateral	nd
Walking aids as needed		nd	cane	cane	nd
Soft brace		a	nd	nd	nd
Alternative and complementary modalities					
Acupuncture		insuff evid			nd
Tai Chi/mind body		insuff evid		nd	nd
Thermal modalities		nd		nd	nd

TENS (if not surgical candidate)	nd	insuff evid		nd	nd
Therapeutic ultrasound		nd	nd	nd	nd
Cognitive-behavioral therapy		nd		nd	nd
Massage	insuff evid	insuff evid			nd
Laser therapy		nd	nd	nd	nd
Balneotherapy		nd	nd	nd	nd
Electromagnetic therapy		nd		nd	nd
Nerve block therapy		nd	nd	nd	nd
extracorporeal shock wave	nd	nd	nd	nd

Colors indicate the direction and strength of recommendations.

Color	Direction	Strength
	For	Strong
	For	Conditional
	For	Weak
	Against	Conditional
	Against	Strong

a Note for DoD bracing: consider soft brace for knee OA, valgus brace for medial compartment OA.

Table 2
Recommendations for the management of hip osteoarthritis

	OARSI	Va/DoD	ACR
Self-management programs and education	Education / Self-mgmt		
Weight Loss (if overweight)			
Exercise		nd	
Low-impact aerobic exercise (aquatic and/or land based)			
Supervised exercise with manual therapy	nd	nd	
Balance		nd	
Manual therapy alone	nd	nd	
Group and home equally effective/individualize	nd	no preference	nd
Consider PT/OT referral			nd
Mobilization and manipulation	nd	nd	nd
Joint support and assistive devices			
Heel wedges (medial or lateral as indicated)	nd	nd	
Walking aids as needed		nd	
Alternative and complementary modalities			
Acupuncture		insuff evid	
Tai Chi/mind body		insuff evid	
Thermal modalities		nd	
TENS (if not surgical candidate)	nd	insuff evid	
Cognitive-behavioral therapy (with or without exercise)		nd	
Massage		insuff evid	
Balneotherapy		nd	nd
Pharmacologic			

Acetaminophen/paracetamol (<4 g/d)			
Oral NSAID		insuff evid	nd
Topical NSAID	nd	insuff evid	nd
Topical capsaicin		insuff evid	nd
Glucosamine and/or chondroitin		insuff evid	
Gastroprotection for high-risk patients (COX2, topicals, add PPI)		a	Discussed, rec as appropriate
Tramadol			
Opioids			
Duloxetine		nd	nd
Diacerhein		nd	nd
Avocado Soybean unsaponifiables		insuff evid	nd
Herbal remedies	Boswellia, curcumin	insuff evid	nd
Vitamins	MSM or vitamin D	insuff evid	Vit D
Intraarticular corticosteroids			
Intraarticular hyaluronic acid			
Intraarticular platelet-rich plasma or growth factors	nd	PRP: insuff evid	nd
DMARDs	nd	nd	nd
Collagen		insuff evid	nd

Colors indicate the direction and strength of recommendations.

Color	Direction	Strength
	For	Strong
	For	Conditional
	For	Weak
	Against	Conditional
	Against	Strong

[a] Consider adding proton pump inhibitor or misoprostol in patients at risk for upper gastrointestinal events who require treatment with NSAIDs or COX-2 inhibitors.

Table 3
Recommendations for the management of hand osteoarthritis

	EULAR	ACR
Education and Self-Management		
Self-management programs and education		
Individualized treatment		Discussed and recommended as appropriate
Exercise	nd	
Range of motion/flexibility		nd
Joint support and assistive devices		
Assistive devices to improve ADLs		nd
Splints for trapeziometacarpal OA		1st CMC / Other hand joints
Alternative and complementary modalities		
Acupuncture	nd	
Thermal modalities	nd	
Cognitive-behavioral therapy (with or without exercise)	nd	
Pharmacologic		
Acetaminophen/paracetamol (<4 g/d)		
Oral NSAID		
Topical NSAID		
Topical capsaicin	Discussed but no recommendation	
Glucosamine	nd	
Chondroitin		
Tramadol	Discussed but no recommendation	
Opioids (refractory pain)	nd	
Duloxetine	nd	
Vitamin D	nd	
Intraarticular corticosteroids		1st CMC
Intraarticular hyaluronic acid	nd	
DMARDs		

Colors indicate the direction and strength of recommendations.

Color	Direction	Strength
	For	Strong
	For	Conditional
	For	Weak
	Against	Conditional
	Against	Strong

across guidelines; these programs typically use a multidisciplinary group-based format addressing skill-building, education about the disease and therapies, joint protection measures, managing weight, and fitness and exercise approaches and goals. It should be noted that often such recommendations were not based on randomized controlled data, but rather driven by the low cost, low harm, and high likelihood of benefit.

Summary Recommendations

Education and self-management constitute a key component of OA management. Referral to self-management programs should be provided, and patients should receive education on OA, management approaches, joint protection strategies, and exercise.

Exercise and weight loss

Exercise and physical activity were consistently and strongly recommended across the guidelines. "Low-impact aerobic exercise" encompasses a variety of more specific recommendations, including aquatic and land-based exercise, and was strongly recommended in 3/6 guidelines (OARSI, ACR/AF, AAOS), especially for knee and hip OA. Exercise was strongly recommended for knee OA in the ESCEO guidelines and as part of a self-management program for knee and hip OA in the VA/DOD guidelines, but no specific exercise recommendations were provided in these guidelines. Balance training was conditionally recommended for knee and hip OA in the ACR/AF guidelines, and neuromuscular training, which includes balance, agility, and coordination exercises, was recommended for knee OA by AAOS. The ACR/AF guidelines provided a conditional recommendation in support of yoga for knee OA due to the lack of high-quality evidence in knee OA. In general, recommendations were made for both supervised (ie, in a physical therapy program) and unsupervised exercise. Generally, there is insufficient evidence to recommend a hierarchy of one type of exercise over another and therefore patient-specific impairments, preferences, and feasibility should be taken into account. Physical therapy referral, as a component of self-management, was conditionally recommended in the VA/DOD guidelines. Range of motion/flexibility exercises was strongly recommended for hand OA in the EULAR guidelines, but overall there was less agreement on the benefits of exercise for hand OA. Weight loss for overweight individuals was consistently recommended for knee and hip OA, with generally moderate to high-quality evidence.

Summary Recommendations

Patients with OA should be advised to engage in regular low-impact aerobic exercise (land or aquatic-based) and to lose weight if overweight. Range of motion/flexibility training should be advised for hand OA. Neuromuscular/balance training and physical/occupational therapy referrals can be considered on an individualized basis. There is no evidence to suggest a hierarchy of one exercise approach over another. Exercise recommendations should be tailored to the individual patient.

Joint support and assistive devices

There was a lack of agreement among guidelines for assistive devices. Kinesiotaping was conditionally recommended for knee and/or first CMC joint OA in the ACR/AF guidelines. In contrast, patellar taping was conditionally not recommended by the OARSI guidelines, due to weak quality of evidence. This modality was not specifically addressed in the other guidelines. Knee braces (including unloader braces with varus force for lateral knee OA or valgus force for medial knee OA) were recommended with moderate quality of evidence in the AAOS guidelines. Tibiofemoral braces were strongly recommended for knee OA, while patellofemoral braces were conditionally recommended for knee OA in the ACR/AF guidelines given variable results across published trials and difficulty some individuals have tolerating these braces. Soft knee braces were conditionally not recommended in the OARSI guidelines but may be considered in some individuals with knee OA according to VA/DOD, though strength of recommendation was not provided. Use of medial and lateral heel wedges was addressed in 3/6 guidelines (OARSI, ACR/AF, AAOS), and supporting evidence was of weak quality. The OARSI guidelines provided a conditional recommendation for heel wedges for knee OA and a conditional recommendation against heel wedges in polyarticular OA. The ACR guidelines provided conditional recommendation against heel wedges for knee and hip OA, and AAOS strongly recommended against the use of lateral heel wedges in knee OA. Walking aids (eg, canes, crutches) were generally recommended as needed for knee and hip OA, with moderate to high-quality evidence for use of canes. Splints for trapeziometacarpal OA were conditionally recommended by EULAR and ACR/AF. First CMC splinting was strongly recommended in the ACR/AF guidelines for hand OA involving the CMC joint.

Summary Recommendations

Walking aids and other assistive devices are recommended on an as-needed basis to improve mobility and activities of daily living in patients with OA. Knee braces, including unloader braces (with varus or valgus force as indicated) and tibiofemoral braces, can be considered for knee OA in appropriate clinical settings based on at least a moderate level of evidence. Patellofemoral knee braces may be considered, but supporting evidence is of weaker quality. Tolerability of knee braces is an issue that should be taken into account. Appropriate fitting and use guided by a physical therapist should be considered when prescribing knee braces. Kinesiotaping may be considered for knee and/or first CMC joint OA, although supporting evidence is limited. Current evidence does not support the use of heel wedges for knee and/or hip OA. Splinting can be considered for patients with hand OA, especially involving the first CMC joint.

Alternative and complementary physical or mind-body modalities

Recommendations for alternative and complementary physical or mind-body treatment approaches were somewhat controversial and differed among societies. Acupuncture was conditionally recommended for patients with knee, hip, and/or hand OA in the ACR/AF guidelines despite limited evidence, given the positive effect of acupuncture for analgesia and low risk of harm. AAOS cited limited evidence for acupuncture in knee OA, and OARSI provided a conditional recommendation against acupuncture for knee, hip, and/or polyarticular OA. Tai chi was strongly recommended for knee and hip OA by ACR/AF and for knee OA by OARSI (also conditionally recommended for hip and polyarticular OA by OARSI). Yoga was conditionally recommended by ACR/AF for knee OA, with a caution for hip OA due to potential issues related to excessive hip abduction.

Thermal modalities were strongly recommended for hip OA by OARSI (conditionally not recommended for knee and polyarticular OA) and conditionally recommended by ACR/AF for knee, hip, and/or hand OA. Transcutaneous electrical nerve stimulation (TENS) was consistently not recommended across guidelines, including in patients who are not surgical candidates. There was insufficient evidence to recommend therapeutic ultrasound, massage therapy, laser therapy, balneotherapy, electromagnetic therapy, nerve block, or extracorporeal shock wave therapy. Cognitive-behavioral therapy (CBT) was conditionally recommended for patients with knee, hip, and/or hand OA by ACR/AF on the basis of data regarding chronic pain management, although further study is needed to better assess the benefit of CBT in OA directly. OARSI provided a conditional recommendation for CBT in patients with knee OA, as well as those with hip and/or polyarticular OA who are frail and/or have cardiovascular or gastrointestinal comorbidities.

Summary Recommendations

Tai chi is recommended for patients with knee, hip, and/or hand OA, with strongest evidence in knee OA. Acupuncture may be considered for knee, hip, and/or hand OA based on potential benefit for analgesia and low risk of harm, although supporting evidence is limited. Thermal modalities may be considered, with strongest evidence in hip OA. Cognitive-behavioral therapy may be helpful for pain reduction and coping and may be considered a component of OA management. TENS is not recommended, including in poor surgical candidates, based on very limited supporting evidence. There is insufficient evidence to recommend therapeutic ultrasound, massage therapy, laser therapy, balneotherapy, nerve block, or extracorporeal shock wave therapy.

Pharmacologic Recommendations

In general, 2 topical agents, 12 classes of oral medications, and 3 types of intraarticular therapies were considered across these guidelines **Table 4**).

Acetaminophen had mixed, primarily weak or conditional recommendations both for and against its use, reflecting the recognition of its poor efficacy but also the need for an alternative for patients in whom other oral agents may not be safe or tolerated. The only guidelines that provided a strong recommendation for acetaminophen were AAOS for the knee and EULAR for the hand.

Oral NSAIDs were generally recommended for all sites of OA, but the strength of recommendations (conditional/weak vs strong) varied among guidelines, primarily reflecting concerns about adverse effects. Some guidelines included the discussion of gastroprotection, but only the OARSI guideline provided a formal GRADE recommendation.

Topical NSAIDs were uniformly strongly recommended for knee OA by all guidelines and were strongly and conditionally recommended for hand OA by EULAR and ACR/AF, respectively, with the strength of recommendation influenced by the practicality of using topical agents on finger joints. Topical NSAIDs were not recommended for the hip due to the deepness of the joint. In contrast, topical capsaicin was conditionally or weakly recommended for knee OA by ACR/AF and VA/DOD, but conditionally recommended against by OARSI. On the hand, EULAR made no recommendations due to challenges with blinding trials, and ACR made a conditional recommend against topical capsaicin primarily due to the logistics of applying the topical agent to the hands and risk of wiping one's eyes, and so forth, which could result in burning sensations elsewhere. Again, this topical agent was not considered for the hip due to the depth of the joint.

Recommendations on the use of tramadol were mixed, either conditionally/weakly against or conditionally/weakly for; this variation was primarily related to the recognition that some patients require an option for pain management when oral NSAIDs are not an option (contraindicated, not tolerated, or ineffective), particularly when considering input from patient panels. In contrast, other forms of opioids were generally recommended against, either strongly or conditionally, due to the recognition of their poor efficacy, substantial adverse effects, and concerns regarding various aspects of the opioid epidemic; dependency was a particular concern voiced by members of the patient panel.

Table 4
Pharmacologic modality recommendations for the management of knee osteoarthritis

	OARSI	VA/DoD	ACR/AF	AAOS	ESCEO
Acetaminophen/paracetamol (<4 g/d)					weak against for long-term use; weak for short-term use
Oral NSAID					
Topical NSAID					
Topical capsaicin				nd	nd
Glucosamine		insuff evid			
Chondroitin		insuff evid			
Combination glucosamine AND chondroitin		insuff evid		nd	weak against short-term use
Gastroprotection for high-risk patients (COX2, topicals, add PPI)		a	Discussed, rec as appropriate	nd	discussed, but no specific rec
Tramadol					
Opioids				nd	
Duloxetine				nd	
Diacerhein		nd	nd	nd	
Avocado Soybean unsaponifiables		insuff evid	nd	nd	
Herbal remedies	Boswellia, Curcuminoid:	insuff evid	nd	turmeric, ginger	nd
Vitamins	MSM, vitamin D	insuff evid	Vitamin D	Vitamin D	nd
Intraarticular corticosteroids					
Intraarticular hyaluronic acid					
Intraarticular platelet-rich plasma or growth factors	nd	PRP: insuff evid stem cells			nd
DMARDs	nd	nd		nd	nd
Collagen		insuff evid			nd

Colors indicate the direction and strength of recommendations.

Color	Direction	Strength
	For	Strong
	For	Conditional
	For	Weak
	Against	Conditional
	Against	Strong

[a] Consider adding proton pump inhibitor or misoprostol in patients at risk for upper gastrointestinal events who require treatment with NSAIDs or COX-2 inhibitors.

Though duloxetine is approved for OA in some countries, there were only conditional or weak recommendations for its use across all guidelines, reflecting general concerns about efficacy and tolerability.

Glucosamine had substantial variation in recommendations across the guidelines. ESCEO made a strong recommendation for the use of glucosamine sulfate in knee OA, whereas OARSI and ACR/AF recommended against its use in knee and hip OA (conditionally and strongly, respectively) and AAOS made a weak recommendation for its use in knee OA. ACR also made a strong recommendation against its use in hand OA, while EULAR made no recommendation due to the lack of placebo-controlled trials conducted in patients with hand OA. Chondroitin, on the other hand, had a conditional recommendation for its use in hand OA by both EULAR and ACR/AF on the basis of a single trial that had low risk of bias, and none of the guidelines recommended chondroitin for other sites with the exception of ESCEO which again provided a strong recommendation for its use in knee OA.

In terms of intraarticular therapies, all of the guidelines recommended intraarticular corticosteroid (IACS) injections for the knee and hip, with most providing a weak or conditional recommendation and ACR/AF providing a strong recommendation; for the hip, the ACR/AF also strongly recommended ultrasound guidance for intraarticular therapy. EULAR made a strong recommendation against IACS for hand OA though commented on its potential use in the case of "clear joint inflammation," whereas ACR provided a conditional recommendation for its use.

In contrast, the recommendations regarding intraarticular hyaluronic acid (IAHA) were quite mixed. For the knee, OARSI, VA/DOD, and ESCEO made weak recommendations for its use, with some specifications, such as if refractory (VA/DoD) or if failed NSAIDs (ESCEO). Both ACR and AAOS provided a conditional recommendation against the use of IAHA for the knee, related to the lack of efficacy data when considering high-quality, low risk of bias trials from well-conducted meta-analyses. IAHA was not recommended for the hip or hand by any of the guidelines. Finally, some guidelines considered intraarticular platelet-rich plasma (PRP) and stem cell therapies. Most guidelines indicated either insufficient evidence to make a recommendation or provided recommendations against their use; the one exception was AAOS which made a weak recommendation for use of intraarticular PRP.

No DMARDs were recommended by any of the guidelines; in fact, there was a strong recommendation against their use by the ACR/AF due to the lack of efficacy demonstrated in numerous trials. Some guidelines considered oral herbal therapies, vitamins, diacerein, avocado soybean unsaponifiables, and collagen. There were mixed recommendations, primarily weak, related to poor or insufficient data, with primarily recommendations against use.

Summary Recommendations

Oral and topical NSAIDs are the pharmacologic agents most recommended for OA, though oral formulations should be avoided in those with contraindications and intolerances, and topical formulations are not appropriate for a deep joint such as the hip. Acetaminophen is no longer considered "first-line" for OA due to its relatively poor efficacy,[12] though it is still an option for those who have contraindications or intolerances to NSAIDs. IACS may be considered, whereas other intraarticular therapies were generally not recommended, or in the case of IAHA, only to be considered if other therapies have failed. Opioids, including tramadol, are generally not recommended, though guidelines did acknowledge that in some cases, such as in instances of contraindications, intolerance to, or inadequate response to NSAIDs, tramadol can be considered for pain relief in the absence of other viable options.

DISCUSSION

The OA treatment guidelines developed by several professional societies over the past few years have numerous similarities in terms of methodology. They have all used GRADE methodology (see Liron Caplan's article, "The GRADE Method," in this issue), included a multidisciplinary team, and for the most part have included patient partners. Clear and transparent management of potential conflicts of interest remain varied, with the ACR/AF having the strongest policy that is in line with recommendations for the development of clinical practice guidelines.

These guidelines also have numerous similarities in their recommendations. They universally recommend education, self-management approaches, and a wide array of physical modalities, with exercise and physical activity (for knee and hip OA primarily) being strongly recommended across all guidelines that considered this modality. For those who are obese or overweight with knee or hip OA, weight loss is also recommended across all guidelines. For pharmacologic therapies, oral and topical NSAIDs remain the primary recommended treatment, though with appropriate caveats regarding contraindications and intolerances. Intraarticular corticosteroids were recommended at varying strengths throughout the guidelines in the recognition of their short-term efficacy. Other intraarticular agents had mixed recommendations. In particular, intraarticular hyaluronic acid had conditional recommendations both for and against its use, reflecting the mixed interpretation of efficacy findings in the context of publication and other biases, and high-quality meta-analyses demonstrating no meaningful efficacy in low risk of bias trials.[13,14] Glucosamine and chondroitin also had mixed levels of recommendations for and against their use, also reflecting the mixed quality of the evidence in the literature with regards to bias.[15]

Why might there be variations in recommendations across guidelines using similar methodologies? First, the systematic literature review is structured with PICO (patient – intervention – comparator – outcome) questions; for a given intervention of interest, what kind of patient, comparator, and outcome is assessed can affect the type of data ultimately available in the evidence report. While the GRADE methodology relies on an evidence report, the quality of evidence can be up- or down-graded based on the risk of bias, which groups may not evaluate in a uniform manner. The voting panel is tasked with interpreting the evidence report as providing evidence "for" or "against" an intervention, and must also decide on the strength of recommendations by taking into account not only the quality of the evidence, but also the balance between potential benefits and potential harms, values and preferences (including feasibility, convenience, and so forth), and cost considerations. Thus, some recommendations could vary by geographic regions due to cost, for example. Another consideration regarding differences across guidelines is that conflicts of interest could certainly influence discussions and ultimately the vote among the expert voting panel.

No clear hierarchy is noted in these guidelines regarding the type of modality to start with (eg, exercise vs NSAIDs, as one example), or for approaches to use first within a modality. For example, there is no hierarchy for the type of exercise to use, and thus patient-centered decision-making can be made to select the right type or combination of exercises. Additionally, one can and should develop an evidence-based individualized multimodal management approach depending on the needs and impairments present in a given patient using the recommended modalities from these guidelines (**Fig. 1**).[16] Thus, there is no longer a treatment pyramid paradigm in managing OA. Instead, one may need to revisit various modalities over time, often in combination, in the course of a given individual's OA journey.

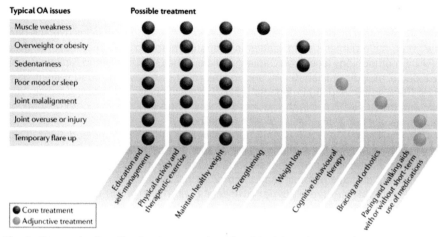

Fig. 1. Core and adjunctive treatment options for OA. A broad range of treatments is recommended by international clinical guidelines for osteoarthritis (OA) management that can be used to address different modifiable risk factors. Education and self-management, therapeutic exercise and physical activity, and maintaining a healthy weight are core treatments for OA. Additional adjunctive treatments can be prescribed depending on the needs of the individual, including the ones shown. Core and adjunctive treatments for OA should be tailored to the individual for optimal personalized care. *From* Bowden JL, Hunter DJ, Deveza LA, Duong V, Dziedzic KS, Allen KD, Chan PK, Eyles JP. Core and adjunctive interventions for osteoarthritis: efficacy and models for implementation. Nat Rev Rheumatol. 2020 Aug;16(8):434-447.

Despite the strong recommendations regarding weight loss, exercise, and physical modalities implemented by physical therapists, lifestyle counseling and referral to physical therapy are substantially underutilized by primary care physicians in the US over the past 15 years, while NSAID and opioid prescriptions have risen over that same period of time.[17] The rise in the prescription of NSAIDs is of concern given that multimorbidity is common in OA,[18] with many such comorbidities being contraindications to NSAIDs. In a population-based Swedish study, ~30% of people with incident knee or hip OA had a contraindication to NSAIDs or a condition that merits precaution with NSAIDs.[19] Furthermore, greater than 20% of those with contraindications to or precautions with NSAIDs were prescribed NSAIDs and were ~30% more likely to be prescribed opioids than those without such contraindications or precautions.[19] People who are obese with OA have a ~2-fold increased risk of being prescribed opioids than those who are normal weight and OA is among the most common reasons for opioid prescription among those who are obese.[20] Thus addressing obesity, referring to physical therapy, and counseling regarding exercise and physical activity (eg, www.cdc.gov/arthritis/interventions/index.htm, https://oaaction.unc.edu/individuals/) are important evidence-based approaches to not only managing OA, but may also help decrease the use of NSAIDs among those with contraindications or precautions to NSAIDs and reduce inappropriate prescription of opioids.

Thus, although professional society treatment guidelines are fairly consistent regarding core recommendations for weight loss, exercise, use of NSAIDs (in the absence of contraindications or precautions), and avoidance of opioids, patterns in clinical practice do not reflect these recommendations. As OA is largely managed in primary care, greater efforts are needed to disseminate and implement evidence-based guidelines into primary care practices.

SUMMARY

The OA treatment guidelines across 6 professional societies are largely concordant with one another. The lack of adequate management for people with OA in the community largely reflects the lack of adequate dissemination and implementation, as well as a paucity of safe and effective pharmacologic options. Patient engagement with culturally appropriate participatory language and counseling regarding weight loss (where appropriate), exercise and physical activity, and greater access to physical modalities such as physical therapy are urgently needed to optimize OA management in the setting of few pharmacologic agents with high-quality evidence to support their use. These guidelines also highlight a major unmet need for developing a broader array of safe, effective therapies and the need for engaging in multimodal care with better targeting of impairments and underlying contributors to symptoms.

CLINICS CARE POINTS

- All patients with OA should receive appropriate education about the disease and management options, as well as counseling regarding self-management approaches.
- Physical modalities including exercise, physical activity, and various physical therapy modalities for knee and hip OA are well-supported by moderate to high-quality evidence. Those who are obese or overweight should be counseled regarding weight-loss approaches.
- There remains a paucity of effective and safe pharmacologic options for the management of OA, with oral and topical NSAIDs being the primary medications recommended.
- Where guidelines are not fully in agreement with one another, that discrepancy usually reflects inadequate strength of evidence supporting efficacy being balanced by the consideration of the therapy when other options are ineffective or cannot be used (eg, contraindications or intolerances). These therapeutic options require engaging in shared decision-making and an individualized management approach.

FUNDING

TN: NIH K24 AR070892, NIH P30 AR072571; AN: NIH P30 AR072580.

DISCLOSURE

C. Overton: none. A.E. Nelson: Pfizer/Lilly. T. Neogi: Novartis, Pfizer/Lilly, Regeneron.

REFERENCES

1. Disease GBD. Injury I, Prevalence C. Global, regional, and national incidence, prevalence, and years lived with disability for 328 diseases and injuries for 195 countries, 1990-2016: a systematic analysis for the Global Burden of Disease Study 2016. Lancet 2017;390(10100):1211–59.
2. Sebbag E, Felten R, Sagez F, et al. The world-wide burden of musculoskeletal diseases: a systematic analysis of the World Health Organization Burden of Diseases Database. Ann Rheum Dis 2019;78(6):844–8.
3. HCUP Fast Stats. Healthcare Cost and Utilization Project (HCUP). Rockville (MD): Agency for Healthcare Research and Quality; 2021. Available at: www.hcup-us. ahrq.gov/faststats/national/inpatientcommonprocedures.jsp?year1=2018& characteristic1=0&included1=1&year2=2008&characteristic2=54&included2=

1&expansionInfoState=hide&dataTablesState=hide&definitionsState=hide&export State=hide.

4. Institute of Medicine (US) Committee on Standards for Developing Trustworthy Clinical Practice Guidelines. In: Graham R, Mancher M, Miller Wolman D, et al, editors. Clinical practice guidelines we can trust. Washington (DC): National Academies Press (US); 2011. https://doi.org/10.17226/13058. Available at: https://www.ncbi.nlm.nih.gov/books/NBK209539/.

5. Kolasinski SL, Neogi T, Hochberg MC, et al. 2019 American College of Rheumatology/Arthritis Foundation Guideline for the Management of Osteoarthritis of the Hand, Hip, and Knee. Arthritis Rheumatol 2020;72(2):220–33.

6. Kolasinski SL, Neogi T, Hochberg MC, et al. 2019 American College of Rheumatology/Arthritis Foundation Guideline for the Management of Osteoarthritis of the Hand, Hip, and Knee. Arthritis Care Res (Hoboken) 2020;72(2):149–62.

7. Bruyere O, Honvo G, Veronese N, et al. An updated algorithm recommendation for the management of knee osteoarthritis from the European Society for Clinical and Economic Aspects of Osteoporosis, Osteoarthritis and Musculoskeletal Diseases (ESCEO). Semin Arthritis Rheum 2019;49(3):337–50.

8. Kloppenburg M, Kroon FP, Blanco FJ, et al. 2018 update of the EULAR recommendations for the management of hand osteoarthritis. Ann Rheum Dis 2019; 78(1):16–24.

9. Bannuru RR, Osani MC, Vaysbrot EE, et al. OARSI guidelines for the non-surgical management of knee, hip, and polyarticular osteoarthritis. Osteoarthritis Cartilage 2019;27(11):1578–89.

10. Brems JH, Davis AE, Clayton EW. Analysis of conflict of interest policies among organizations producing clinical practice guidelines. PLoS one 2021;16(4): e0249267.

11. Bunzli S. Pearls: How (and Why) to use participatory language when communicating with patients about osteoarthritis. Clin Orthop Relat Res 2021;479(8): 1669–70.

12. da Costa BR, Reichenbach S, Keller N, et al. Effectiveness of non-steroidal anti-inflammatory drugs for the treatment of pain in knee and hip osteoarthritis: a network meta-analysis. Lancet 2017;390(10090):e21–33.

13. Rutjes AW, Juni P, da Costa BR, et al. Viscosupplementation for osteoarthritis of the knee: a systematic review and meta-analysis. Ann Intern Med 2012;157(3): 180–91.

14. Johansen M, Bahrt H, Altman RD, et al. Exploring reasons for the observed inconsistent trial reports on intra-articular injections with hyaluronic acid in the treatment of osteoarthritis: meta-regression analyses of randomized trials. Semin Arthritis Rheum 2016;46(1):34–48.

15. Wandel S, Juni P, Tendal B, et al. Effects of glucosamine, chondroitin, or placebo in patients with osteoarthritis of hip or knee: network meta-analysis. BMJ 2010; 341:c4675.

16. Bowden JL, Hunter DJ, Deveza LA, et al. Core and adjunctive interventions for osteoarthritis: efficacy and models for implementation. Nat Rev Rheumatol 2020;16(8):434–47.

17. Khoja SS, Almeida GJ, Freburger JK. Recommendation Rates for Physical Therapy, Lifestyle Counseling, and Pain Medications for Managing Knee Osteoarthritis in Ambulatory Care Settings: A Cross-Sectional Analysis of the National Ambulatory Care Survey (2007-2015). Arthritis Care Res (Hoboken) 2020;72(2): 184–92.

18. Swain S, Sarmanova A, Coupland C, et al. Comorbidities in osteoarthritis: a systematic review and meta-analysis of observational studies. Arthritis Care Res (Hoboken) 2020;72(7):991–1000.

19. Neogi T, Dell'isola A, Englund M, et al. Frequent Use of Prescription Oral NSAIDs Among People with Knee or Hip Osteoarthritis Despite Contraindications to or Precautions with NSAIDs [abstract]. Arthritis Rheumatol 2021;73(suppl 10). Available at: https://acrabstracts.org/abstract/frequent-use-of-prescription-oral-nsaids-among-people-with-knee-or-hip-osteoarthritis-despite-contraindications-to-or-precautions-with-nsaids/.

20. Stokes A, Lundberg DJ, Sheridan B, et al. Association of Obesity With Prescription Opioids for Painful Conditions in Patients Seeking Primary Care in the US. JAMA Netw Open 2020;3(4):e202012.

Treatment Guidelines in Gout

Allan C. Gelber, MD, MPH, PhD

KEYWORDS

- Gout • Guidelines • Treatment • Target

KEY POINTS

- When treating acute gout with colchicine, low-dose dosing is the only way to go.
- Treat-to-target is key to reduce the frequency of flares, diminish tophaceous deposits, arrest radiographic damage, and improve quality of life.
- For severe refractory tophaceous gout, pegloticase is a viable therapeutic option.
- When evaluating a patient at the office, at an urgent care facility, or as a hospitalized inpatient, the comorbidity profile, including the heightened risk of cardiovascular morbidity and mortality associated with gout, should be considered.
- An enhanced understanding of uric acid crystal–mediated activation of the inflammasome complex, inflammatory cytokines, and mediators of neutrophil excitation informs the biological basis for novel agents to enter the gout therapeutic armamentarium.
- The potential (but as yet not proven) role for dietary modification and exercise enhancement to improve gout activity should be kept in mind.

INTRODUCTION

Acute and chronic gout, the prototypic microcrystalline arthropathy, is a disorder that all health care providers, including physicians, nurses, and allied health professionals alike, are exposed to in the course of their education, training, and careers, given the high prevalence of gout in society. An illustrative gout-related clinical interaction with a colleague appears in Appendix 1. Moreover, this clinical reality is relevant in both the ambulatory and inpatient settings. Adults may present with severe joint warmth, redness, swelling, and pain that necessitates hospitalization, in the throes of an acute gout attack.[1] Oftentimes it is acute gout, in and of itself, that prompts admission to the medicine service. Alternatively, acute gout may rear its head as a consequence and secondary complication of a distinct pathophysiologic process that initially prompted the hospitalization (eg, myocardial infarction, congestive heart failure, sepsis, an elective operative procedure).

Johns Hopkins University School of Medicine, Mason F. Lord Building, Center Tower, Suite 4100, 5200 Eastern Avenue, Baltimore, MD 21224, USA
E-mail address: agelber@jhmi.edu

Rheum Dis Clin N Am 48 (2022) 659–678
https://doi.org/10.1016/j.rdc.2022.04.003
0889-857X/22/© 2022 Elsevier Inc. All rights reserved.

In recent decades the incidence and prevalence of gout has been increasing, both nationally within the United States and internationally across the globe.[2,3] There are several explanations to account for this observation. First, as gout occurrence increases with each advancing decade of life, a concomitant increase in average life span observed in the closing decades of the twentieth century, and now 22 years into the new millennium, expands the number of persons at risk to develop gout. Second, major comorbid disorders associated with gout incidence are themselves increasing, including hypertension, hyperlipidemia, overweight and obesity, chronic kidney disease, and the metabolic syndrome, each an increasingly prevalent disorder in contemporary society.[4,5] The steady increase in these disorders, among a growing number of persons in mid and late adult life, contribute to the escalating prevalence of gout. Consequently, as we each age, and particularly as growing numbers of women enter the postmenopausal phase of life when gout incidence exponentially increases, we face a heightened risk to develop gout.[6]

Although gout can and does occur in the pediatric age population, including in preadolescence, notably among children born with inherited disorders of purine metabolism, the focus of this review and of the gout guidelines promulgated by the internal medicine and rheumatology societies is on the adult age spectrum of gout.

HISTORY

When the *New England Journal of Medicine* published a review article a half century ago on the treatment of gout, the therapeutic options described for the treatment of *acute gouty arthritis* consisted of colchicine, nonsteroidal anti-inflammatory drugs [NSAIDs] (notably indomethacin and phenylbutazone), and corticosteroid therapy.[7] With regard to colchicine dosing it was delineated that "no more than 12 consecutive tablets should be given under any circumstance." Furthermore, at that time, steroid therapy was not particularly in vogue, describing how "occasionally, a very brief course of ACTH or corticosteroid treatment is useful for achieving defervescence of severe and refractory gout."[7]

At the time, control of serum urate levels in the chronic management of gout consisted of 2 approaches. The first was induction of uricosuria by blocking the renal tubular reabsorption of uric acid. This strategy entailed use of either probenecid or sulfinpyrazone. The alternate approach amounted to antagonism of the xanthine oxidase enzyme in the purine metabolic pathway. For this purpose, allopurinol was the drug of choice and had come into common practice in the preceding decade.[8] Even at that point in time, decades ago, the control of serum urate was highlighted as a major priority in the management of gout. The overall goal was to achieve a "sustained reduction of the serum urate concentration to values below 6 mg per 100 mL."[7]

A quarter century later an updated review on the management of gout was again published in the *Journal*.[9] As before, the 3 frontline agents to manage acute gout arthritis remained colchicine, NSAIDs, and corticosteroids. Reflecting that 25-year evolution in thinking, however, the review indicated that "colchicine is less favored now than in the past because its onset of action is slow and it invariably causes diarrhea." Colchicine dosing was still described with a total dose of 8 mg (equivalent to 16 0.5-mg tablets administered every 2 hours). It was also noteworthy that intravenous colchicine remained a viable therapeutic option, a practice that has since entirely vanished. NSAIDs continued to play a prominent role in the treatment algorithm. However, the upside of NSAIDs was counterbalanced by their known propensity to induce gastrointestinal symptoms and renal dysfunction, both notably problematic among the elderly. In contrast to the early 1970s' review, the 1996 article now emphasized the wide applicability of corticosteroid agents including availability in several preparations (intra-articular injection, systemic oral prednisone, intramuscular corticotropin or triamcinolone, and intravenous methylprednisolone). In addition, several agents were listed as options to lower serum urate concentrations including probenecid, sulfinpyrazone, salicylate, diflunisal, benzbromarone, and continued use of allopurinol. The review also emphasized the necessity to include either colchicine or an NSAID agent as a prophylactic approach to prevent acute gout from flaring during initiation of a urate-lowering agent, an approach that became common clinical practice.

In this sequence of reviews in the *New England Journal of Medicine* regarding gout management, a major development that preceded the 2011 article on gout was the immunologic discovery that monosodium urate crystals initiate acute inflammation by engaging the caspase-1-activating NLRP3 (cryopyrin) inflammasome.[10] Inflammasome activation in turn results in activation of intracellular interleukin-1β, with heightened levels downstream of interleukin-1 and interleukin-18. Appreciation of this molecular mechanism enabled an improved understanding of how uric acid crystals trigger an acute inflammatory response characteristic of gout flares.

This finding also furnished a biological basis for the series of published reports using interleukin-1 antagonists as therapeutic agents in the management of acute gout. Three such products have come to market and antagonize various components of interleukin-1-mediated inflammation. Specifically, canakinumab is a direct antagonist to interleukin-1β release, rilonacept antagonizes circulating levels of interleukin-1, and anakinra inhibits the interleukin-1 receptor.[11–13] Each has been studied in the treatment of gout. However, gout is not a Food and Drug Administration [FDA]-approved indication for their use. Yet, this line of enquiry piques one's interest and fascination with potential additional agents that may come to market, including modification of terminal complement pathway components, inhibition of leukotrienes, and inhibitors of neutrophil recruitment, to control gout-related inflammation.

BACKGROUND

A seemingly unfortunate commentary on the current state of affairs in gout care, nationally and globally, is the suboptimal delivery of effective treatment in practice.[14] Far too often patients with gout are not treated in a timely fashion to relieve their acute flares, not appropriately dosed to optimize their path to recovery, and do not have their urate-lowering agents titrated to minimize, if not abolish, gout recurrence.[15–17] Such efforts in both the inpatient and ambulatory settings to manage gout are similarly poorly delivered. Several explanations may contribute to these shortcomings, including inadequate access to the health care system and inadequate knowledge and familiarity among health care providers at properly prescribing and tracking the efficacy of gout medications, particularly relevant when it comes to urate-lowering therapy.

Both urate-lowering strategies (xanthine oxidase inhibition and uricosuria) require vigilance for potential drug-related toxicity. Moreover, those with more severe gout are apt to harbor comorbid disorders, which in turn pose relative contraindications to the effective and safe use of gout prophylaxis; this is particularly applicable with coexistent chronic kidney disease, which enhances the risk to develop gout while also representing a major risk factor for iatrogenic injury, particularly noteworthy with allopurinol. As such, even though allopurinol has been the standard urate-lowering agent for more than a half century, it is recognized that health care providers and gout specialists alike do not escalate the dose of allopurinol with sufficient regularity to bring persons with recurrent and disabling gout under adequate control.[14–17] It is for all these reasons that the guidelines reviewed in this article are particularly informative, and relevant, to the care of the ever-increasing number of persons afflicted with gout.

American College of Physicians Gout Clinical Practice Guideline

The clinical report, entitled "Management of Acute and Recurrent Gout: A Clinical Practice Guideline from the American College of Physicians," was published online in 2016.[18]

The American College of Physicians (ACP) guidelines were based on critical analysis of randomized controlled trials, systematic reviews, and large observational studies published between 2010 and 2016. The purpose was to provide guidance on the management of acute and chronic gout in the adult age population. The guidelines committee used the GRADE approach (Grading of Recommendations Assessment, Development and Evaluation) based on available published evidence. Four specific recommendations resulted, as depicted below in **Box 1**:

Observations on American College of Physicians gout guideline

It has been suggested that the ACP guidelines are in conflict with those disseminated by the rheumatology societies. A fundamental difference between them is the absence of a treat-to-target focus among the 4 ACP recommendations. In contrast, the European League Against Rheumatism, (EULAR) and American College of Rheumatology (ACR) both place a preeminent role in defining 6 mg/dL (360 μmol/L) as the target level below which clinicians and patients should maintain serum uric acid levels, while working in concert to realize improved clinical, radiographic, and functional outcomes.[19,20] By treating to target, the frequency of acute incapacitating gout flares can be meaningfully reduced and quality restored in the lives of those with gout.

Rather than being contradictory guideline statements, the apparent discrepancy may reflect the landscape of patient communities the 2 societies each serve. In the case of the ACP, in making a recommendation to internists, it is absolutely critical to articulate the foremost priority to initiate effective gout therapy in the throes of an acute gout attack. It is also a priority to initiate urate-lowering therapy for those persons with a high frequency of recurrent gout attacks that greatly interfere with their vocational and leisure time activities and overall quality of life. However, it is not necessary to commence urate-lowering therapy for all patients with gout. The general internist will care for a broad spectrum of disease severity, including those with mild and moderate gout. Consequently, those persons with a first gout attack, or with distinctly infrequent gout flares, do not necessitate treatment beyond acute flare management.

Box 1
American College of Physicians Clinical Practice Guideline

Recommendation 1: ACP recommends clinicians choose corticosteroids, nonsteroidal anti-inflammatory drugs, or colchicine to treat patients with acute gout.

Recommendation 2: ACP recommends that clinicians use low-dose colchicine when using colchicine to treat acute gout.

Recommendation 3: ACP recommends against initiating long-term urate-lowering therapy in most patients after first gout attack or in patients with infrequent attacks.

Recommendation 4: ACP recommends that clinicians discuss benefits, harms, costs, and individual preferences with patients before initiating urate-lowering therapy, including concomitant prophylaxis in patients with recurrent gout attacks.

At the same time, and reflecting the focus of the EULAR and ACR guidelines (addressed later herein), the rheumatology community frequently serves a population, referred by the internist, that constitutes the more severe end of the gout disease spectrum. In caring for patients with more frequent attacks, those with a greater proportion of tophaceous deposits, and those with radiographic evidence of erosive gout arthropathy, the EULAR and ACR guidelines inform the rheumatology community on how to optimize outcomes for this patient population based on the current state of evidence derived from the published literature.

Were the frontline primary care provider to achieve desirable gout disease control, referral to the rheumatologist would likely not follow. Yet, it is through the rheumatologist's lens, in being asked to evaluate patients with refractory disease, or those patients for whom a meaningful improvement in disease control or in quality of life has not yet been achieved, that a compelling need to articulate a quantitative (treat-to-target) measure is in order. This is the premise for an easily defined and measurable target serum uric acid level, below the solubility of urate in plasma, and emphasizes the key role hyperuricemia plays at instigating gout flares. Moreover, in clinical studies, achievement of a target level serves as a key outcome measure related to improved disease control. In practice, serum uric acid constitutes an objective parameter to assess whether a given patient's therapeutic regimen is on track. When the target level has not yet been achieved, there is a clear message to the patient and provider alike to jointly address regimen adherence and to consider further dose adjustment.

It is also important to note that sufficient published data were not available to comment within the ACP guideline on subgroups defined by gender, acute episode, history of gout, HLA-B*5801 genotype category, tophaceous status, or comorbidities.[18]

Importantly, high-quality evidence was identified which indicated that colchicine reduces pain among those with acute gout attacks. Furthermore, it was recognized that colchicine is associated with adverse gastrointestinal side effects including nausea, vomiting, abdominal cramps, and pain. With use of NSAIDs, gastrointestinal adverse effects are similarly recognized, including from minor dyspepsia to serious and life-threatening perforations, ulcers, and bleedings. NSAIDs may also induce renal insufficiency.

Colchicine. For decades, colchicine has been a critical element in the treatment algorithm to manage acute gout. Yet, colchicine dosing has changed dramatically over the last 20 years. The new dosing algorithm is consequently reflected in the treatment guidelines. Previously, generations of medical students and medicine house officers alike were routinely instructed to manage an acute gout flare by prescribing 2 colchicine tablets at time equals 0, then continue with 1 additional (0.5- or 0.6-mg) tablet at 1- to 2-hour intervals until (1) the acute gout flare was aborted, (2) the patient experienced diarrhea, or (3) a predetermined maximum number of tablets had been administered.[7,9] In contrast to that traditional dosing schedule for colchicine, now termed *high-dose colchicine*, the new *low-dose colchicine* approach consists of 2 tablets at time equals 0, and then a third and final tablet administered 1 hour later.[21] This approach is a dramatically different dosing schedule for acute gout management yet one with demonstrated equal efficacy to the former algorithm.

In a high-impact paper published in 2010, the old dosing algorithm of colchicine was examined in a randomized, double-blind, placebo-controlled parallel group study.[21] The 3 arms of the study were low-dose colchicine (1.8 mg over 1 hour), high-dose colchicine (4.8 mg over 6 hours), and placebo.[21] A favorable response to the primary end point, being 50% or greater reduction in pain at 24 hours, without use of rescue medication, was observed in a comparable proportion of those assigned to the low- and high-dose colchicine groups, and in substantially fewer in the placebo group. The therapeutic benefit of colchicine was clinically and statistically significant compared with placebo. Furthermore, a most informative finding was that the low-dose colchicine group experienced a similar adverse event profile as that of the placebo group. In contrast, high-dose colchicine was associated with a higher frequency of diarrhea and vomiting. Consequently, this trial has completely changed the paradigm of colchicine dosing in the management of acute gout over the subsequent decade.

Finally, it is also important to note, as is stated in the introduction to the ACP guideline, that the contemporary management of gout includes both pharmacologic and nonpharmacologic approaches. The latter may focus on dietary and lifestyle management, including weight loss and exercise. Yet, we should not lose sight of the fact that although such a nonpharmacologic strategy seems appealing, and that benefit may accrue to affected persons with gout who are able to achieve weight reduction and/or a higher exercise level, or both, substantive published evidence to support such an intervention is currently lacking.

2016 European League Against Rheumatism Recommendations

In 2016, EULAR (renamed European Alliance of Associations for Rheumatology) convened a steering group to update its earlier 2006 recommendations for the management of gout.[22] The steering committee recognized the importance of having clear diagnostic criteria to improve the delivery of gout care, a worldwide concern.[14,17] Notable deficiencies in this domain include (1) delays in the diagnosis of gout, (2) inadequate utilization of well-accepted therapies in the management of acute and chronic gout, and (3) inadequate titration of urate-lowering agents to derive their full clinical benefit. Alternatively stated, although viable, generally well-tolerated treatment strategies exist, they are too often suboptimally implemented in practice to prevent the sequelae of tophaceous gout, erosive gout, and quality of life-limiting gout.

The task force consisted of rheumatologists, general practitioners, musculoskeletal radiologists, as well as patients and methodologists from 12 European countries. Updated published reports, from the calendar period of 2005 to 2013, including from MEDLINE, EMBASE, and Cochrane Library databases, were reviewed.[22] The task force unanimously voted to modify its earlier, 2006, set of recommendations, to reflect updated published evidence. An important feature of the 2016 guideline was that "wherever possible the recommendation should take the form of a clear active recommendation specific to a particular clinical situation."

Importantly the 2016 EULAR update disseminated 3 overarching principles, listed in **Box 2**, and 11 recommendations (detailed in Appendix 2)[19].

Observations on European League Against Rheumatism Gout Recommendations
Over the decade of time between publication of the 2006 and the subsequent 2016 EULAR gout treatment guidelines, the options for gout therapy had changed rather dramatically. The guideline authors indicated that, in 2006, allopurinol, for all intent and purposes, was the main agent used to lower serum uric acid levels. Over the subsequent 10-year interval, several new drugs either became available in common practice or were at advanced stages of development, including febuxostat, pegloticase, inhibitors of interleukin-1, and lesinurad. The authors further noted that dosing schedules for conventional drugs, including both colchicine and allopurinol, had also been modified during that interval decade. Furthermore, a third notable development was

---

Box 2
2016 European League Against Rheumatism Recommendations

Overarching principle A: Every person with gout should be fully informed about the pathophysiology of the disease, the existence of effective treatments, associated comorbidities, and the principles of managing acute attacks and eliminating urate crystals through lifelong lowering of serum uric acid level to less than the target level.

Overarching principle B: Every person with gout should receive advice regarding lifestyle, including weight loss, as appropriate, and avoidance of alcohol (particularly beer and spirits) as well as avoidance of sugar-sweetened drinks, heavy meals, and excessive intake of meat and seafood. Low-fat dairy products should be encouraged. Regular exercise should be advised.

Overarching principle C: Every person with gout should be systematically screened for associated comorbidities and cardiovascular risk factors, including renal impairment, coronary heart disease, heart failure, stroke, peripheral arterial disease, obesity, hyperlipidemia, hypertension, diabetes, and smoking. These comorbidities should be addressed as an integral part of the management of gout.

---

heightened awareness of an adverse cardiovascular morbidity and mortality profile associated with antecedent gout.

There are several important issues raised by the EULAR guidelines that warrant elaboration. First, there are many aspects about lifestyle, including diet, exercise, weight management, and the spectrum of comorbidities that are relevant to gout care. As outlined in overarching principle A this lifestyle dimension ought to be integrated as an essential component of communication between providers and persons with gout. Consequently, this emphasis within the EULAR recommendations on the fundamental importance of health care provider-patient communication amounts to a breath of fresh air. This principle is broadly applicable in the evaluation and management of a full spectrum of medical disorders, across internal medicine and rheumatology. The EULAR guidelines specifically emphasize the importance of meaningful communication in the management of gout.

Next, overarching principle B emphasizes that it is not only what we eat but also what we drink that makes a difference in the development and management of gout. There were a series of critical epidemiologic observational reports emanating from the Health Professionals Follow-up Study that furnished exquisitely detailed and highly informative insights into the relationship of specific elements of the human diet to incident gout.[23] These reports highlighted not only the relationship of meat consumption to incident gout but also the specific components of meat, such as beef versus pork versus poultry. In addition, this seminal report indicated that consumption of not only crustacean seafood but also of canned tuna is associated with increased gout incidence.[23] Moreover, from these observational data we also learn how consumption of low-fat dairy, and not all (and any) dairy, is specifically related to a reduction in incidence of gout.

Moreover, from the same longitudinal cohort we are informed that weight reduction is associated with a diminished incidence of gout.[24] Further, not all types of alcohol contribute the same risk of gout.[25] Notably, consumption of beer is associated with the highest incidence of gout, in a dose-response association. Next come spirits, which harbor an intermediate risk between that of beer and wine. However, wine consumption itself is not associated with an increase in incidence of gout.

The third overarching principle relates to a substantial increase in epidemiologic studies in the last 2 decades highlighting the association of various comorbid disorders with gout incidence and prevalence. As such, principle C emphasizes the intersection of risk factors common to both atherosclerotic cardiovascular disease and gout.[4] These conditions include overweight, obesity, hypertension, chronic kidney disease, diabetes mellitus, hyperlipidemia, and the metabolic syndrome. Intriguingly, principle C takes this concept to an entirely new level by articulating a highly lofty goal that a diagnosis of gout should alert, flag, and heighten the awareness of the treating provider to carefully consider and screen for incident cardiovascular disease.[26–28]

2020 American College of Rheumatology Guideline for the Management of Gout.

In 2020, the ACR published an updated guideline for the management of gout; a previous ACR guideline had been published 8 years earlier.[29,30] Importantly, the 2020 update adhered to the college's guideline development process, integrating the GRADE methodology. This approach enables the reader to quickly grasp the strength of the evidence because each recommendation is designated with 1 of 4 distinct and mutually exclusive categories, being "strongly recommend," "conditionally recommend," "strongly recommend against," and "conditionally recommend against." A particular benefit of this approach was to yield a set of guidelines that emphasizes actionable gout management items in clinical practice. Several key components of the ACR 2020 guidelines are listed in **Box 3** (these guidelines are detailed in Appendix 3).

Observations on American College of Rheumatology Gout Guideline

It is noteworthy that the patient panel members, critically involved in the development of this guideline, conveyed that whereas they were initially hesitant to commence ULT agents, after they had experienced improvement in disease control they became strong advocates for early initiation of these medications.

Febuxostat. In the years just preceding the 2006 EULAR guidelines, febuxostat was investigated and determined to be a viable second xanthine oxidase inhibitor in the prevention of recurrent gout.[31] Febuxostat was therefore integrated into the 2012 ACR guidelines, has become entrenched into the current armamentarium, and appears prominently in the 2016 EULAR and 2020 ACR guidelines. Previously, for at least 40 years, allopurinol was the prototype and lone member of this pharmacologic category. By inhibiting xanthine oxidase, dosing with allopurinol interrupted the purine metabolic pathway such that hypoxanthine is not converted to xanthine, xanthine is not converted to urate, and a lowering in serum uric acid level is achieved.

A seminal article published in 2005 examined febuxostat, as a novel xanthine oxidase inhibitor, among 762 patients with gout.[31] There were 3 arms to the clinical trial consisting of (1) allopurinol dosed at 300 mg once daily, (2) low-dose febuxostat at 80 mg once daily, and (3) high-dose febuxostat at 120 mg, also dosed once daily. The duration of treatment was a full year or 52 weeks. Importantly, prophylaxis against acute gout flares, following the initiation of these 2 xanthine oxidase inhibitors, was undertaken through the first 8 weeks of the study. The primary end point was achievement of a serum uric acid concentration of less than 6 mg/dL (360 μmol/L); secondary end points included incident rates of gout flares and tophaceous deposit surface area size. It is important to note that in the United States, the FDA-approved doses of febuxostat are either 40 mg or 80 mg orally once daily.

Ultimately, the trial demonstrated that both doses of febuxostat were more efficacious than the fixed (standard) dose of allopurinol at achieving the serum uric acid target. In contrast, the impact on gout flare activity and on tophaceous burden size was comparable in all 3 groups. It is notable that treatment with febuxostat over allopurinol is particularly attractive among persons with gout who harbor comorbid

---

Box 3
American College of Rheumatology 2020 Guideline

Initiating ULT for patients with gout is *strongly recommended* for those who have (1) 1, or more, subcutaneous tophus, (2) evidence of radiographic damage attributable to gout, or (3) frequent gout flares defined as 2 or more annual flares.

Initiating ULT is *conditionally recommended against* in patients with asymptomatic hyperuricemia.

Starting treatment with low-dose allopurinol at or less than 100 mg daily, and even lower in patients with CKD (stage 3, 4 or 5), and febuxostat ($\leq$40 mg daily) with subsequent dose titration over starting at a higher dose, is *strongly recommended.*

Administering concomitant anti-inflammatory prophylaxis therapy (eg, colchicine, nonsteroidal anti-inflammatory drug, prednisone/prednisolone) over no anti-inflammatory prophylaxis therapy is *strongly recommended.*

Achieving and maintaining an SUA target of less than 6 mg/dL over the use of no target is *strongly recommended* for all patients receiving ULT.

Testing for the HLA-B*5801 allele before starting allopurinol is *conditionally recommended* for patients of Southeast Asian descent (eg, Han Chinese, Korean, Thai) and for African American patients, over not testing for the HLA-B*5801 allele.

Switching to pegloticase over continuing current ULT is *strongly recommended* for patients with gout for whom xanthine oxidase inhibitor treatment, uricosurics, and other interventions have failed to achieve the target serum uric acid level, and who continue to have frequent gout flares ($\geq$2 flares per year) or who have nonresolving subcutaneous tophi.

---

moderate-to-severe chronic kidney disease; febuxostat is predominantly metabolized by the liver, whereas allopurinol is primarily metabolized in the kidney.

Over the many decades that allopurinol has been the predominant agent used to lower SUA, this agent has not been clearly implicated with a heightened risk of adverse cardiovascular morbidity and mortality. That having been said, in the high-profile clinical trial of febuxostat, when compared to allopurinol, there were 4 deaths observed during the follow-up period. Notably, all 4 were among patients assigned to the febuxostat arm of the trial; none were observed in the allopurinol group.[27,31] This observation prompted awareness and emphasized the importance of postmarketing pharmacoepidemiology to ascertain if an adverse cardiovascular profile would ensue as febuxostat was disseminated into the general population.

A subsequent report examined cardiovascular outcomes, among patients with established gout and prevalent cardiovascular disease, assigned to either febuxostat or allopurinol in a multicenter double-blind trial.[28] The primary endpoint was a composite index of cardiovascular death, nonfatal myocardial infarction, nonfatal stroke, or unstable angina with urgent revascularization. There were a total of 6190 patients assigned to these 2 therapeutic options followed for a median of 32 months. All-cause mortality and cardiovascular mortality were 22% higher in the febuxostat group compared with allopurinol (hazard ratio 1.22; 95% confidence interval 1.01–1.47). The hazard ratio for the outcome of cardiovascular death alone was 1.35 (1.03–1.73). Consequently, it remains important to be cautious in the prescription of febuxostat to those patients with gout with concomitant coronary atherosclerosis and established coronary heart disease.

Pegloticase. A decade ago, in 2011, a landmark clinical trial documented the experience of 225 patients from 56 rheumatology practices in the United States,

Canada, and Mexico, each experiencing severe gout, allopurinol intolerance or refractoriness, and a measured serum uric acid level greater than 8 mg/dL.[32] The patients were randomized to receive 12 biweekly intravenous dosings, containing either pegloticase at each infusion, pegloticase alternating with placebo at successive infusions, or placebo infusions only. The primary outcome measure was achievement of a serum uric acid level less than 6 mg/dL, the traditional target SUA level. In the pooled analysis, 42% of those assigned to biweekly pegloticase infusions achieved the primary end point compared with none in the placebo arm. There were 7 deaths observed, 4 among those receiving pegloticase and 3 among those receiving placebo. This novel recombinant mammalian uricase, designed to replace the absent expression of the urate oxidase (uricase) gene in primate mammals, not only resulted in a marked reduction in serum uric acid levels but also led to improved disease control and markedly enhanced resolution of tophaceous deposits. This was a transformative report and introduced a new entrant into the armamentarium of gout therapeutics.

Drug-drug interaction.. Next, an important principle articulated in these guidelines is vigilance for potential drug-drug interaction associated with colchicine therapy. Specifically, in the context of gout and related comorbid disorders, and the common concurrent prescriptions of both colchicine and a statin agent, the latter to treat hyperlipidemia and atherosclerotic cardiovascular disease, there is a reasonable high probability to develop drug-related toxicity. Notably, both these agents act as substrates and inhibitors of the cytochrome P450 (CYP3A4 and P-glycoprotein) enzymatic pathways. Consequently, drug-induced toxicity may follow from the interaction between these 2 agents, thereby resulting in the development of myopathy and even severe rhabdomyolysis.[33]

HLA-B*5801. An additional substantive development in the last 15 years was the identification of genetic susceptibility to develop allopurinol toxicity, including the allopurinol hypersensitivity syndrome and related Stevens-Johnson syndrome and toxic epidermal necrolysis.[34] The genetic variant HLA-B*5801 confers a predisposition to allopurinol-related adverse cutaneous reactions, particularly in the Han Chinese population. Consequently, allopurinol should either be avoided or dosed at particularly low levels (eg, 50 mg daily, or 100 mg thrice weekly), and then be carefully titrated upward with serial monitoring in these patients. More recently, the feasibility of screening for HLA-B*5801 within the United States has demonstrated this approach to be cost-effective.[35] Undertaking such testing among Asians and African Americans, but not among Caucasians or Hispanics, was cost-effective. Furthermore, review of Medicaid data from hospitalization across the United States demonstrated that the risk of developing severe cutaneous adverse reactions attributed to allopurinol was greatest among blacks, Asian, and Native Hawaiian/Pacific Islanders, particularly among older women.[36]

Losartan. An interesting aspect of gout therapy, and particularly relevant to the comorbidity profile that gout keeps, is the notion that choice of antihypertensive agent may favorably affect gout risk. In a United Kingdom general practice database, among 24,768 persons who developed gout, compared with 50,000 matched controls, the risk of incident gout varied by choice of antihypertensive medication.[37] Notably, losartan, but not other angiotensin II receptor blockers, was associated with a reduced risk of developing gout compared with diuretics, angiotensin-converting enzyme inhibitors, and beta-blockers.

Diet. Finally, there have been a few published studies that have focused on the consumption of vitamin C and cherries, and dietary modification, in relation to gout risk.[38–44] To date, these studies have primarily focused on the association of dietary composition with levels of serum uric acid rather than with gout disease activity. These findings suggest that elements in our diet may have a favorable impact on gout. However, these findings are only supportive of this notion, at present, and are not conclusive. Nevertheless, it is conceptually appealing to consider that what we eat and what we drink can one day favorably affect gout incidence, and possibly gout recurrence, at the population level.

SUMMARY

In this article, updated gout guidelines from the ACP, EULAR, and ACR are each reviewed in detail, with a focus on highlighting to the reader key elements of the published literature in gout that support the evolution of these guidelines and recommendations over time. The reader, whether of a primary internal medicine or rheumatology background, and whether currently undertaking or beyond their years of training, will be informed on the key elements of these various professional societies in the management of gout. Increased familiarity and proficiency in this domain is ultimately indispensable to improve clinically relevant outcomes and quality of life among those persons affected by gout.

CLINICS CARE POINTS

- When caring for a patient with repeated flares of acute gouty arthritis, initiate urate lowering therapy [ULT] to reduce the risk of gout recurrence.
- Titrate urate lowering therapy to achieve a target serum uric acid level below 6 mg/dL (or 360 μmol/L).
- Allopurinol is the first-line drug of choice ULT agent; commence at a low dose, especially among persons with chronic kidney disease, and titrate upwards to achieve target.
- Conceptualize a gout clinical encounter as an opportunity to screen for associated comorbidities and cardiovascular risk factors.

FUNDING

Dr. Gelber received support from NIH/NIAMS RO1 AR073178.

CONFLICTS OF INTEREST

The author had full access to the article and a singular role in article writing; the author has nothing to disclose.

REFERENCES

1. Neogi T. Clinical practice: gout. N Engl J Med 2011;364(5):443–52.
2. Juraschek SP, Miller ER 3rd, Gelber AC. Body mass index, obesity, and prevalent gout in the United States in 1988-1994 and 2007-2010. Arthritis Care Res (Hoboken) 2013;65(1):127–32.
3. Dehlin M, Jacobsson L, Roddy E. Global epidemiology of gout: prevalence, incidence, treatment patterns and risk factors. Nat Rev Rheumatol 2020;16(7): 380–90.

4. Juraschek SP, Kovell LC, Miller ER, et al. Dose-response association of uncontrolled blood pressure and cardiovascular disease risk factors with hyperuricemia and gout. PLoS One 2013;8(2):e56546.

5. Juraschek SP, Kovell LC, Miller ER 3rd, et al. Association of kidney disease with prevalent gout in the United States in 1988-1994 and 2007-2010. Semin Arthritis Rheum 2013;42(6):551–61.

6. Arromdee E, Michet CJ, Crowson CS, et al. Epidemiology of gout: is the incidence rising? J Rheumatol 2002;29(11):2403–6.

7. Goldfinger SE. Treatment of gout. N Engl J Med 1971;285(23):1303–6.

8. Rundles RW, Metz EN, Silberman HR. Allopurinol in the treatment of gout. Ann Intern Med 1966;64(2):229–58.

9. Emmerson BT. The management of gout. N Engl J Med 1996;334(7):445–51.

10. Martinon F, Pétrilli V, Mayor A, et al. Gout-associated uric acid crystals activate the NALP3 inflammasome. Nature 2006;440(7081):237–41.

11. So A, De Meulemeester M, Pikhlak A, et al. Canakinumab for the treatment of acute flares in difficult-to-treat gouty arthritis: Results of a multicenter, phase II, dose-ranging study. Arthritis Rheum 2010;62(10):3064–76.

12. Terkeltaub R, Sundy JS, Schumacher HR, et al. The interleukin 1 inhibitor rilonacept in treatment of chronic gouty arthritis: results of a placebo-controlled, monosequence crossover, non-randomised, single-blind pilot study. Ann Rheum Dis 2009;68(10):1613–7.

13. McGonagle D, Tan AL, Shankaranarayana S, et al. Management of treatment resistant inflammation of acute on chronic tophaceous gout with anakinra. Ann Rheum Dis 2007;66(12):1683–4.

14. Singh JA, Hodges JS, Toscano JP, et al. Quality of care for gout in the US needs improvement. Arthritis Rheum 2007;57(5):822–9.

15. Doherty M, Jansen TL, Nuki G, et al. Gout: why is this curable disease so seldom cured? Ann Rheum Dis 2012;71(11):1765–70.

16. Juraschek SP, Kovell LC, Miller ER 3rd, et al. Gout, urate-lowering therapy, and uric acid levels among adults in the United States. Arthritis Care Res (Hoboken) 2015;67(4):588–92.

17. Kuo CF, Grainge MJ, Mallen C, et al. Rising burden of gout in the UK but continuing suboptimal management: a nationwide population study. Ann Rheum Dis 2015;74(4):661–7.

18. Qaseem A, Harris RP, Forciea MA. Clinical Guidelines Committee of the American College of Physicians. Management of Acute and Recurrent Gout: A Clinical Practice Guideline From the American College of Physicians. Ann Intern Med 2017;166(1):58–68.

19. Richette P, Doherty M, Pascual E, et al. 2016 updated EULAR evidence-based recommendations for the management of gout. Ann Rheum Dis 2017;76(1):29–42.

20. FitzGerald JD, Dalbeth N, Mikuls T, et al. 2020 American College of Rheumatology guideline for the management of gout. Arthritis Care Res (Hoboken) 2020;72(6):744–60.

21. Terkeltaub RA, Furst DE, Bennett K, et al. High versus low dosing of oral colchicine for early acute gout flare: Twenty-four-hour outcome of the first multicenter, randomized, double-blind, placebo-controlled, parallel-group, dose-comparison colchicine study. Arthritis Rheum 2010;62(4):1060–8.

22. Zhang W, Doherty M, Bardin T, et al. EULAR evidence based recommendations for gout. Part II: Management. Report of a task force of the EULAR Standing

Committee for International Clinical Studies Including Therapeutics (ESCISIT). Ann Rheum Dis 2006;65(10):1312–24.

23. Choi HK, Atkinson K, Karlson EW, et al. Purine-rich foods, dairy and protein intake, and the risk of gout in men. N Engl J Med 2004;350(11):1093–103.

24. Choi HK, Atkinson K, Karlson EW, et al. Obesity, weight change, hypertension, diuretic use, and risk of gout in men: the health professionals follow-up study. Arch Intern Med 2005;165(7):742–8.

25. Choi HK, Atkinson K, Karlson EW, et al. Alcohol intake and risk of incident gout in men: a prospective study. Lancet 2004;363(9417):1277–81.

26. Gelber AC, Klag MJ, Mead LA, et al. Gout and risk for subsequent coronary heart disease. The Meharry-Hopkins Study. Arch Intern Med 1997;157(13):1436–40.

27. Gelber AC. Febuxostat versus allopurinol for gout. N Engl J Med 2006;354(14): 1532–3.

28. White WB, Saag KG, Becker MA, et al. Cardiovascular safety of febuxostat or allopurinol in patients with gout. N Engl J Med 2018;378(13):1200–10.

29. Khanna D, Fitzgerald JD, Khanna PP, et al. 2012 American College of Rheumatology guidelines for management of gout. Part 1: systematic nonpharmacologic and pharmacologic therapeutic approaches to hyperuricemia. Arthritis Care Res (Hoboken) 2012;64(10):1431–46.

30. Khanna D, Khanna PP, Fitzgerald JD, et al. 2012 American College of Rheumatology guidelines for management of gout. Part 2: therapy and antiinflammatory prophylaxis of acute gouty arthritis. Arthritis Care Res (Hoboken) 2012;64(10): 1447–61.

31. Becker MA, Schumacher HR Jr, Wortmann RL, et al. Febuxostat compared with allopurinol in patients with hyperuricemia and gout. N Engl J Med 2005; 353(23):2450–61.

32. Sundy JS, Baraf HS, Yood RA, et al. Efficacy and tolerability of pegloticase for the treatment of chronic gout in patients refractory to conventional treatment: two randomized controlled trials. JAMA 2011;306(7):711–20.

33. Schwier NC, Cornelio CK, Boylan PM. A systematic review of the drug-drug interaction between statins and colchicine: Patient characteristics, etiologies, and clinical management strategies. Pharmacotherapy 2022;42(4):320–33. https:// doi.org/10.1002/phar.2674, the paper has now been published. Should list CITATION for this article just like all the others - to be uniform! allan In this issue.

34. Hung SI, Chung WH, Liou LB, et al. HLA-B*5801 allele as a genetic marker for severe cutaneous adverse reactions caused by allopurinol. Proc Natl Acad Sci U S A 2005;102(11):4134–9.

35. Jutkowitz E, Dubreuil M, Lu N, et al. The cost-effectiveness of HLA-B*5801 screening to guide initial urate-lowering therapy for gout in the United States. Semin Arthritis Rheum 2017;46(5):594–600.

36. Keller SF, Lu N, Blumenthal KG, et al. Racial/ethnic variation and risk factors for allopurinol-associated severe cutaneous adverse reactions: a cohort study. Ann Rheum Dis 2018;77(8):1187–93.

37. Choi HK, Soriano LC, Zhang Y, et al. Antihypertensive drugs and risk of incident gout among patients with hypertension: population-based case-control study. BMJ 2012;344:d8190.

38. Juraschek SP, Miller ER 3rd, Gelber AC. Effect of oral vitamin C supplementation on serum uric acid: a meta-analysis of randomized controlled trials. Arthritis Care Res (Hoboken) 2011;63(9):1295–306.

39. Zhang Y, Neogi T, Chen C, et al. Cherry consumption and decreased risk of recurrent gout attacks. Arthritis Rheum 2012;64(12):4004–11.

40. Gelber AC, Solomon DH. If life serves up a bowl of cherries, and gout attacks are "the pits": implications for therapy. Arthritis Rheum 2012;64(12):3827–30.

41. Dalbeth N, Ames R, Gamble GD, et al. Effects of skim milk powder enriched with glycomacropeptide and G600 milk fat extract on frequency of gout flares: a proof-of-concept randomised controlled trial. Ann Rheum Dis 2012;71(6):929–34.

42. Juraschek SP, McAdams-Demarco M, Gelber AC, et al. Effects of Lowering Glycemic Index of Dietary Carbohydrate on Plasma Uric Acid Levels: The OmniCarb Randomized Clinical Trial. Arthritis Rheumatol 2016;68(5):1281–9.

43. Juraschek SP, Gelber AC, Choi HK, et al. Effects of the Dietary Approaches to Stop Hypertension (DASH) Diet and Sodium Intake on Serum Uric Acid. Arthritis Rheumatol 2016;68(12):3002–9.

44. Rai SK, Fung TT, Lu N, et al. The Dietary Approaches to Stop Hypertension (DASH) diet, Western diet, and risk of gout in men: prospective cohort study. BMJ 2017;357:j1794.

APPENDIX 1

CASE STUDY

In the course of preparing this review, I was approached by a colleague in the context of her general medicine practice, as follows:

I am caring for an older old male patient with stage 3 CKD, HTN, DM2 controlled on oral agents, obesity who has had 2-3 gout flares over the last year. I would like to start allopurinol to help prevent additional flares. Serum uric acid is ~ 9 mg/dL. I am a bit stumped about what to do with the prophylactic anti-inflammatory therapy during the first 3-6 months of treatment. With his CKD, I worry about low dose NSAIDs for that long of a period and he has not tolerated colchicine in the past (diarrhea). I read that you can do "low dose" prednisone which is worrisome in someone with DM and HTN and I also found an article that suggested that if you start at a low dose and increase slowly that you may be able to do without a prophylactic anti-inflammatory? What has been your experience? I appreciate any advice you have.

This query is quite reminiscent of others that arise each year. The approach to this narrative, and to the care of persons with gout, more broadly, is addressed directly in the guidelines and pages of this review.

Allan

APPENDIX 2

2016 EUROPEAN LEAGUE AGAINST RHEUMATISM RECOMMENDATIONS

Recommendations

(#1) Acute gout flares should be treated urgently. Patient should be educated to self-medicate at the first warning symptoms;

(#2) Frontline therapy for acute gout flares consists of colchicine and/or an NSAID, oral corticosteroid and/or synovial fluid aspiration and intraarticular injection of a corticosteroid agent; Colchicine and NSAIDs should be avoided in patients with chronic kidney disease. Colchicine should not be given to patients receiving strong P-glycoprotein and/or CYP3A4 inhibitors such as cyclosporine or clarithromycin.

(#3) If faced with a contraindication to the three frontline therapeutic agents (detailed immediately above), then an interleukin-1 inhibitor drug should be considered a viable option; Such IL-1 inhibitors should only be initiated in the absence of a concurrent infection; further, ULT should be adjusted to achieve the uricaemia target following IL-1 blocker treatment for flare.

(#4) Gout prophylaxis therapy should be actively discussed with and fully explained to the patient. Prophylaxis is recommended during the first six month of ULT. The primary prophylactic option is colchicine, at a dose of 0.5-1 mg /day, a dose that should be reduced among those with renal impairment. In the case of chronic kidney disease or with co-administration of a statin agent, one need be aware of potential neurotoxicity and/or muscular toxicity with prophylactic colchicine. Concurrent administration of colchicine with a strong P-glycoprotein and/or CYP3A4 inhibitor should be avoided.

(#5) Initiation of a ULT agent should be considered and discussed with every patient with a definite diagnosis of gout from the first presentation. Urate lowering therapy is indicated for all persons with recurrent gout flares (≥2/year), tophi, urate arthropathy and/or renal stones. Initiation of ULT is recommended close to the time of the first diagnosis of gout among persons who develop gout at a young age (<40 years), with hyperuricemia >8 mg/dL; 480 μmol/L), and / or those persons with comorbidities (e.g., CKD, hypertension, ischemic heart disease, congestive heart failure). Patients with gout should receive full information and be fully involved in decision-making concerning the use of ULT.

(#6) For persons received ULT, serum uric acid level monitoring is a critical component of care. A target goal is < 6 mg/dL (360 μmol/L). An even lower SUA target < 5 mg/dL (300 μmol/L) is appropriate to facilitate faster dissolution of crystals among those with severe gout (defined as those with tophi, chronic arthropathy, frequent attacks) until total crystal dissolution and resolution of attack is achieved.

(#7) ULT should be commenced at a low dose, then titrate upward until the SUA target is achieved. SUA < 6mg/dL (360 μmol/L) should be maintained lifelong.

(#8) Among patients with normal renal function, allopurinol is recommended as first-line therapy. Allopurinol ought to be started at the low dose of 100 mg/ day, then up titrated by 100 mg increments every 2-4 weeks, if required, to achieve the uricaemic target. When the SUA is not achieved with appropriate dosing of allopurinol, allopurinol should be switched to febuxostat or to a uricosuric agent, or combined with a uricosuric agent. Febuxostat and a uricosuric agent are to be considered viable alternatives if the use of dose of allopurinol is not well tolerated.

(#9) In the setting of renal impairment, the allopurinol maximum dosage should be adjusted to creatinine clearance. If the SUA target cannot be achieved at this dose, the patient should be switched to febuxostat or to benzbromarone, with or without allopurinol, except among persons with eGFR <30 mL/min.

(#10) Pegloticase is indicated for persons with crystal-proven gout who harbor severe debilitating chronic tophaceous gout and poor quality of life, when the target SUA cannot be achieved with any other oral ULT agent (or combination of agents) at its (their) maximum dose.

(#11) When gout occurs in a patient receiving a loop or thiazide diuretic, consider an alternate non-diuretic agent, including losartan or calcium channel blocker for hypertension.

APPENDIX 3

AMERICAN COLLEGE OF RHEUMATOLOGY GUIDELINE.

INDICATIONS FOR PHARMACOLOGIC ULT

Initiating ULT for patients with gout is *strongly recommended* for those who have (A) ≥1 subcutaneous tophus; (B) evidence of radiographic damage attributable to gout; OR (C) frequent gout flares defined as 2 or more annual flares.

Initiating ULT is *conditionally recommended* for patients who have previously experience >1 flare but have infrequent flares (less than 2/year).

Initiating ULT is *conditionally recommended* **against** in patients with gout experiencing their first gout flare.

Initiating ULT is *conditionally recommended* for patients with comorbid moderate-to-severe CKD who harbor serum uric acid [SUA] concentrations >9 mg/dL or have urolithiasis.

Initiating ULT is *conditional recommendation* **against** in patients with asymptomatic hyperuricemia.

RECOMMENDATIONS FOR CHOICE OF INITIAL ULT FOR PATIENTS WITH GOUT.

Treatment with allopurinol as the preferred first-line agent, over other ULT's, this is *strongly recommended* for all patients, including those with moderate-to-severe CKD (stages 3, 4 or 5).

The choice of either allopurinol or febuxostat over probenecid is *strongly recommended* for patients with moderate-to-severe CKD.

The choice of pegloticase as a first-line therapy is *strongly recommended* **against.**

Starting treatment with low-dose allopurinol at or below 100 mg daily, and even lower in patients with CKD (stage 3, 4 or 5), and febuxostat (≤ 40 mg daily) with subsequent dose titration over starting at a higher dose of *strongly recommended.*

Starting treatment for low-dose probenecid (500 mg once daily or twice daily) with subsequent dose titration over starting at a higher dose is *conditionally recommended.*

Administering concomitant anti-inflammatory prophylaxis therapy (e.g., colchicine, nonsteroidal anti-inflammatory drug, prednisone/prednisolone) over no anti-inflammatory prophylaxis therapy is *strongly recommended.*

Continuing concomitant anti-inflammatory prophylaxis therapy for 3-6 months over less than 3 months, with ongoing evaluation and continued prophylaxis as needed if the patient continues to experience gout flares, is *strongly recommended.*

TIMING OF ULT INITIATION

When the decision is made that ULT is indicated while the patient is experiencing a gout flare, starting ULT during the gout flare over starting ULT after the gout flare has resolved is *conditionally recommended.*

A treat-to-target management strategy that includes ULT dose titration and subsequent dosing guided by serial serum uric acid [SUA] measurements to achieve a target SUA, over a fixed-dose ULT strategy, is *strongly recommended* for all patients receiving ULT.

Achieving and maintaining an SUA target of less than 6 mg/dL over the use of no target is *strongly recommended* for all patients receiving ULT.

Delivery of an augmented protocol of ULT dose management by nonphysician providers to optimize the treat-to-target strategy that includes patient education, shared decision-making, and treat-to-target protocol is *conditionally recommended* for all patients receiving ULT.

DURATION OF ULT

Continuing ULT indefinitely over stopping ULT is *conditionally recommended.*

Allopurinol

Testing for the HLA–B*5801 allele prior to starting allopurinol is *conditionally recommended* for patients of Southeast Asian descent (e.g., Han Chinese, Korean, Thai) and for African American patients, over not testing for the HLA–B*5801 allele.

Universal testing for the HLA–B*5801 allele prior to starting allopurinol is *conditionally recommended against* in patients of other ethnic or racial background over testing for the HLA–B*5801 allele.

Starting allopurinol in daily doses of ≤100 mg (and lower doses in patients with CKD) is *strongly recommended* over starting at a higher dose.

Allopurinol desensitization is *conditionally recommended* for patients with a prior allergic response to allopurinol who cannot be treated with other oral ULT agents.

Febuxostat

Switching to an alternative oral ULT agent, if available and consistent with other recommendations in this guideline, is *conditionally recommended* for patients taking febuxostat with a history of CVD or a new CVD-related event.

Uricosurics

Checking urinary uric acid is *conditionally recommended against* for patients considered for or receiving uricosuric treatment.

Alkalinizing the urine is *conditionally recommended against* for patients receiving uricosuric treatment.

WHEN TO CONSIDER CHANGNING ULT STRATEGY

Switching to a second xanthine oxidase inhibitor agent over adding a uricosuric agent is *conditionally recommended* for patients taking their first xanthine oxidase inhibitor, who have persistently high serum uric acid concentrations (>6 mg/dL) despite maximum-tolerated or FDA-indicated dosing, and who have continued frequent gout flares (>2 flares per year) OR who have nonresolving subcutaneous tophi.

Switching to Pegloticase over continuing current ULT is *strongly recommended* for patients with gout for whom xanthine oxidase inhibitor treatment, uricosurics, and other interventions have failed to achieve the target serum uric acid level, and who continue to have frequent gout flares (≥2 flares per year) or who have nonresolving subcutaneous tophi

Switching to pegloticase over continuing current ULT is *strongly recommended against* for patients with gout for whom xanthine oxidase inhibitor treatment, uricosurics, and other interventions have failed to achieve the serum uric acid target but who have infrequent gout flares AND no tophi.

GOUT FLARE MANAGEMENT

Using colchicine, NSAIDs or glucocorticoids (oral, intraarticular, or intramuscular) as appropriate first-line therapy for gout flares over IL-1 inhibitors or adrenocorticotropic hormone (ACTH) is *strongly recommend* for patients experiencing a gout flare.

Given similar efficacy and a lower risk of adverse effects, low-dose colchicine over high-dose colchicine is *strongly recommended* when colchicine is the chosen agent.

Using topical ice as an adjuvant treatment over no adjuvant treatment is *conditionally recommended* for patients experiencing a gout flare.

Using an IL-1 inhibitor over no therapy (beyond supportive/analgesic treatment) is *conditionally recommended* for patients experiencing a gout flare for whom the above anti-inflammatory therapy is either ineffective, poorly tolerated, or contraindicated.

Treatment with glucocorticoids (intramuscular, intravenous, or intraarticular) over IL-1 inhibitors or ACTH is *strongly recommended* for patients who are unable to tolerate oral medications.

MANAGEMENT OF LIFESTYLE FACTORS

Limiting alcohol intake is *conditionally recommended* for patients with gout, regardless of disease activity.

Limiting purine intake is *conditionally recommended* for patients with gout, regardless of disease activity.

Limiting high-fructose corn syrup is *conditionally recommended* for patients with gout, regardless of disease activity.

Using a weight loss program (no specific program endorsed) is *conditionally recommended* for those patients with gout who are overweight / obese, regardless of disease activity.

Adding vitamin C supplementation is *conditionally recommended* **against** for patients with gout, regardless of disease activity.

MANAGEMENT OF CONCURRENT MEDICATIONS

Switching hydrochlorothiazide to an alternate antihypertensive when feasible is *conditionally recommended* for patients with gout, regardless of disease activity.

Choosing losartan preferentially as an antihypertensive agent when feasible is *conditionally recommended* for patients with gout, regardless of disease activity.

Stopping low-dose aspirin (for patients taking this medication for appropriate indications) is *conditionally recommended* **against** for patients with gout, regardless of disease activity.

Adding or switching cholesterol-lowering agents to fenofibrate is *conditionally recommended* **against** for patients with gout, regardless of disease activity.

Treatment Guidelines in Rheumatoid Arthritis

Jasvinder A. Singh, MBBS, MPH[a,b,c,*]

KEYWORDS

- Rheumatoid arthritis • Treatment guidelines • Recommendations
- Disease-modifying antirheumatic drug • DMARD • Biologic • Methotrexate

KEY POINTS

- Disease-modifying antirheumatic drug (DMARD) treatment should be initiated early in all patients with rheumatoid arthritis.
- The therapeutic dose of methotrexate, 15 to 25 mg weekly, should be used for at least 2 to 3 months, before deeming it an inadequate response, unless intolerable adverse events occur at this dose (using it with folic acid).
- Treatment escalation with addition of other conventional synthetic, biologic, or targeted synthetic DMARDs is indicated if the patient does not achieve low disease activity or remission with methotrexate alone.
- Frequent disease activity monitoring and treatment escalation is needed in rheumatoid arthritis, until the disease can be treated to a target of low disease activity or remission.

THE PURPOSE OF TREATMENT GUIDELINES

Treatment guidelines are frequently formulated to help a busy clinician to make treatment decisions for frequently encountered clinical situations. An obvious question is how does this integrate with the current practice, providers knowledge and experience, and specific situations for a given individual patient? For health conditions and diseases, where the advances are gradual and treatment options are few, decisions with regards to treatment can be boiled down to a simple treatment flowchart or a quick discussion to choose from the few (two or three) most common medications. However, in diseases that are an active hotbed of research and new treatment such decisions are complex and could benefit from the availability of treatment guidelines.

[a] Medicine Service, VA Medical Center, 700 19th Street South, Birmingham, AL 35233, USA; [b] Department of Medicine at the School of Medicine, University of Alabama at Birmingham, 510 20th Street South, Birmingham, AL 35294-0022, USA; [c] Department of Epidemiology, University of Alabama at Birmingham School of Public Health, 1665 University Boulevard, Ryals Public Health Building, Birmingham, AL 35294-0022, USA
* University of Alabama at Birmingham, Faculty Office Tower 805B, 510 20th Street South, Birmingham, AL 35294-0022.
E-mail address: Jasvinder.md@gmail.com
Twitter: @jassingh00 (J.A.S.)

Rheum Dis Clin N Am 48 (2022) 679–689
https://doi.org/10.1016/j.rdc.2022.03.005
0889-857X/22/Published by Elsevier Inc.

rheumatic.theclinics.com

There have been a lot of advances in the treatment of rheumatoid arthritis (RA) in the last three decades. Several new medications and even new classes of drugs have been launched and are available for use in common practice. With rapidly evolving knowledge, and new short- and long-term data from clinical trials and real-world clinical registries, it is challenging to have an updated synthesis of knowledge for a common practitioner. Therefore, the availability of comprehensive systematic literature review, its evaluation by subject experts, and the formulation of evidence-based treatment guidelines can serve as a useful tool for use by a busy practitioner taking care of complex patients with RA.

Several treatment guidelines are available for treatment of RA and range from a comprehensive document that covers not only the treatment of RA but also its management in the presence of other comorbid conditions,[1–4] to a focused guidance for treat-to-target strategy,[5] management of these medications during pregnancy[6] or in the perioperative period,[7] or for monitoring their use.[8] This article reviews the history and main aspects of various RA treatment guidelines, and main findings, as they apply to common clinical situations, and the minor differences between guidelines. These RA treatment guidelines are also referred to as recommendations, guideline, or guidelines. In general, the intent and purpose are that these documents should serve as a useful tool for treatment management rather than be proscriptive.

HISTORY AND THE SCOPE OF KEY RHEUMATOID ARTHRITIS GUIDELINES

I focus primarily on the guidelines that were published in the last 5 to 10 years because the evolution of knowledge in this area of RA therapeutics is fast and many treatment guidelines that are much older may not be completely relevant in the current time.

For the purposes of ease of discussion, I focus primarily on the 2021 American College of Rheumatology (ACR) guideline,[1] the 2019 European League Against Rheumatism (EULAR; now the European Alliance of Associations for Rheumatology) guideline,[2] the 2019 National Institute of Health and Care Excellence (NICE) guideline,[3] and the 2019 Canadian Rheumatology Association (CRA) guideline.[4] Because the CRA guideline was based on review of other guidelines rather than a systematic review of the literature, I only discuss it where appropriate. Most of the focus of the remaining article is key recommendations from ACR, EULAR, and NICE. **Table 1** shows the scope and the main topics covered in the most recent version of each of these guidelines. A recently published review summarized the key similarities and differences between the ACR and EULAR guideline processes.[9] A recent systematic review of RA guidelines provides a summary analysis of 21 guidelines.[10]

The 2021 ACR treatment guideline[1] updates the previous versions of the RA treatment guidelines from 2015,[11] 2012,[12] and 2008.[13] These previous versions have independent sections on laboratory monitoring, tuberculosis screening, management of high-risk comorbidities, and vaccination, much of which is still pertinent.[11–13] The systematic review of the literature for these evidence-based guidelines is provided as supplementary material with each publication.

EULAR published its most recent guideline in 2019,[2] which updates the previous versions from 2016,[14] 2013,[15] and 2010.[16] Systematic reviews that form the basis of these evidence-based guidelines are provided as accompanying articles to the guideline, usually in the same issue of the journal. For example, the systematic review for the 2019 EULAR guideline is available.[17]

NICE published its guidance in 2019,[3] alongside reviews on specific medications.[18–23] This updates its previous guideline published in 2018.[24] The British Society of Rheumatology (BSR) also previously published the 2008 guideline.[25] NICE

Table 1
Scope and the main topics covered in each of the RA treatment guidelines

Guideline	Topics Covered	SLR	Evidence Rating	Types of Recommendations
2021 ACR[1]	All DMARDs; glucocorticoids; high-risk populations	Yes	GRADE certainty: very low, low, moderate, or high	Strong or conditional
2019 EULAR[2]	All DMARDs; glucocorticoids	Yes	Oxford Center for EBM for the level of evidence, 1a to 5; level of agreement from 0 to 10	Strength, A to D
2020 NICE[3]	All DMARDs; glucocorticoids	Yes	GRADE or GRADE-CERQual (for individual or synthesized studies)	Integrates GRADE with a review of the quality of cost-effectiveness studies. Uses the wording of recommendations to reflect the strength of the evidence
2011 CRA[4]	All DMARDs; glucocorticoids	No[a]	Levels of evidence, I (meta-analyses or trial) to IV (expert opinion)	AGREE score for each subsection of the guideline

Abbreviations: AGREE, appraisal of guidelines for research and evaluation; CERQual, Confidence in the Evidence from Reviews of Qualitative research; DMARD, disease-modifying antirheumatic drug; GRADE, grading of recommendations, assessment, development, and evaluations; SLR, systematic literature review.

[a] Systematic review of guidelines (not of the primary literature) was done to identify, appraise, synthesize, and adapt international guidelines for use in Canadian health care context.

pathways will not be updated after December 31, 2021 and this site will be withdrawn in spring 2022.

TREATMENT OF DISEASE-MODIFYING ANTIRHEUMATIC DRUG–NAIVE PATIENT WITH RHEUMATOID ARTHRITIS

One of the most common treatments given to disease-modifying antirheumatic drug (DMARD)-naive patients with RA is methotrexate (MTX). MTX is the current gold standard first-line treatment of RA and is a prototype conventional synthetic DMARD (csDMARD). It is available in multiple formulations including oral and subcutaneous injections. MTX is one of the anchor drugs that is frequently used as monotherapy or as part of a combination therapy to improve signs and symptoms of RA. Most treatment guidelines, including the EULAR, ACR, BSR, and CRA guidelines, recommend MTX as the first-line treatment. This is based on the documented efficacy of MTX for controlling sign of symptoms of RA; high rates of reduction of disease activity with MTX; and the evidence from recent trials of direct comparison of targeted synthetic (tsDMARD) or biologic DMARDs with MTX in the treatment-naive patient population, where comparable rates of response were usually evident. These were frequently numerically similar to and only sometimes lower than those for the comparator biologic or tsDMARD. Alternative csDMARDs are leflunomide, sulfasalazine, and hydroxychloroquine.

Few adverse events require laboratory monitoring (transaminitis, leukopenia, bone marrow suppression) and these and others (gastrointestinal, alopecia, fatigue) can lead to MTX dose reduction (in conjunction with use of 1–5 mg daily folic acid) or discontinuation. This leads to treatment escalation with addition of or substitution with other DMARDs. Inadequate response to MTX is another common reason for treatment escalation, with addition of or switching to other DMARDs, in MTX-treated patients.

The 2019 NICE guideline recommends starting treatment with one conventional DMARD rather than a combination DMARD therapy, based on the evidence of the lack of superiority for the latter approach.[3] This guideline also indicated that there was no difference in the effectiveness of MTX, leflunomide, and sulfasalazine as monotherapy and the costs were similar; hydroxychloroquine was reserved for people with mild or palindromic disease.

The 2021 ACR treatment guideline recommended the following in DMARD-naive people with moderate to high disease activity RA: MTX monotherapy over hydroxy-chloroquine, sulfasalazine, leflunomide, biologic DMARD, or tsDMARD monotherapy; and MTX monotherapy over combination therapy that includes another csDMARD, tsDMARD, or biologic DMARD.[1] In people with low disease activity, hydroxychloro-quine was recommended over other csDMARD, sulfasalazine recommended over MTX, and MTX recommended over leflunomide. Short-term glucocorticoids may be used in combination with this treatment.

The 2019 EULAR treatment guideline recommended starting MTX as monotherapy and combining it with short-term glucocorticoids as needed in DMARD-naive pa-tients.[2] In people with contraindication for MTX, the recommendation was to start leflunomide or sulfasalazine, in combination with short-term glucocorticoids.

Both the 2021 ACR and the 2019 EULAR treatment guidelines provided details with regards to MTX dosing (at least 15 mg weekly within 4–6 weeks of treatment initiation), the route of administration (oral first, but try subcutaneous if oral administration is not optimally effective), and folic acid supplementation. Both also acknowledge the role of short-term glucocorticoids in the initial treatment of RA.

Key Clinical Points for Conventional Synthetic Disease-Modifying Antirheumatic Drug–Naive Patient with Rheumatoid Arthritis

1. An early DMARD treatment initiation is extremely important for RA management and should be a goal achieved in most patients.
2. Always try the therapeutic dose of MTX, 15 to 25 mg weekly, oral or subcutane-ously, for 2 to 3 months, before deeming it an efficacy-failure, or inadequate response, unless intolerable adverse events prohibit the trial.
3. Most gastrointestinal, and rarely, fatigue adverse events, are partially or completely reversible/avoidable with an increase in folic acid dose to 5 mg daily (or rarely, fo-linic acid rescue), and/or MTX dose reduction.
4. Like many other RA DMARDs, the peak efficacy for MTX is usually noted between 3 and 6 months of treatment, especially with a dose taper-up regimen, and even in patients without dose taper-up.
5. Aiming for a treat-to-target approach, in some patients, with a shared decision-making, treatment may already be escalated before the 6-month treatment time-point.

6. Treat-to-target with minimization of harms and intolerable adverse events should be a goal in these patients.
7. At least low RA disease activity should be achieved, if not remission. The optimal period at which this should be achieved may differ based on patient preferences and values, current disease activity, and possibly the presence of prognostic factors.
8. Short-term glucocorticoids are an important adjunct to treatment for achieving initial disease control or managing flares, and this must be balanced against the adverse events associated with their long-term use.

TREATMENT OF CONVENTIONAL SYNTHETIC DISEASE-MODIFYING ANTIRHEUMATIC DRUG–EXPERIENCED PATIENT WITH RHEUMATOID ARTHRITIS

In patients who do not initially respond to csDMARD, treatment escalation is recommended to reduce disease activity. This is achieved by addition of or substitution with another csDMARD, biologic DMARD, or tsDMARD. The current evidence and experience suggest that the addition of DMARDs may be a more effective strategy compared with substitution. However, step-up therapy with addition of DMARDs is associated with greater patient medication burden. Therefore, shared decision-making is critical.

Various guidelines have a range of recommendations with regards to what the second step in the treatment should be. There are several potential reasons for various guidelines to come up with different recommendations. They may be viewing different evidence, because the major guidelines are never done at the same time, and the strength of evidence can change. The method of synthesis of evidence many be different, including the method used to ascertain the strength or certainty of evidence (see **Table 1**). The guidelines may be formulated with different geographic areas and countries/continents in mind, and the availability of medications can differ. The weighting of actual drug cost, type of cost (patient out of pocket vs insurance payer vs government), and patient values and preferences in developing the recommendations may be different. Finally, the importance of financial conflicts and its management for guideline developers may differ among various guidelines. Many of these factors can potentially impact the recommendation decision-making process and contribute to the differences in the final product.

The EULAR guideline recommends that such decision be based on the presence of poor prognostic factors, such as seropositivity, early joint damage, high disease activity, and failure of two or more csDMARDs. For people with poor prognostic factors, the recommendation is to add a biologic DMARD or a tsDMARD to the current csDMARD. The guideline places both medication options, biologic DMARD versus tsDMARD, as reasonable treatments for this group of patients. For people without poor prognostic factors, the recommendation is to switch to or add another csDMARD.

However, the 2021 ACR guideline recommends the addition of biologic DMARD or tsDMARD to the current MTX over triple DMARD therapy (MTX, sulfasalazine, and hydroxychloroquine as the common example) in people with moderate-high disease activity despite MTX monotherapy. In patients who are MTX-naive but csDMARD-experienced, MTX monotherapy was recommended over a combination therapy with biologic DMARD, or tsDMARD.

The 2018 NICE guideline recommends adding another csDMARD to the current csDMARD, rather than switching to another csDMARD for people with active disease despite csDMARD monotherapy. The 2018 NICE guideline does not make recommendation for a specific csDMARD at treatment initiation or treatment escalation but recognized that MTX is the most used csDMARD.

Key Clinical Points for Conventional Synthetic Disease-Modifying Antirheumatic Drug–Experienced Patient with Rheumatoid Arthritis

1. In csDMARD-experienced patients with RA with active disease despite the current use of MTX, the recommendation is step-up therapy with the addition of another DMARD. Various guidelines differ with regards to whether this should be another csDMARD versus biologic DMARD, or tsDMARD.
2. A treat-to-target strategy is highly desirable in these patients who have not tried a biologic DMARD, or tsDMARD. At least low RA disease activity should be achieved, if not remission.
3. Simply continuing or escalating glucocorticoids is not the preferred approach for management of moderate-high disease activity; such increase in disease activity must be managed by step-up DMARD therapy (see point 1 for details).

TREATMENT OF BIOLOGIC OR TARGETED SYNTHETIC DISEASE-MODIFYING ANTIRHEUMATIC DRUG–EXPERIENCED PATIENT WITH RHEUMATOID ARTHRITIS

A variety of options may be available at this treatment decision time point. People may have previously experienced tumor necrosis factor (TNF)-biologic, non-TNF-biologic, or tsDMARD in various combinations. Various guidelines differ with regards to recommendations.

The 2021 ACR guidelines recommended that in people who have active disease despite the current treatment with a biologic DMARD or tsDMARD, the treatment should be switched to a biologic DMARD, or tsDMARD of a different class rather than switching to the same class.

The 2019 EULAR guideline recommends changing the biologic DMARD or tsDMARD to a different or same class if the RA is active despite adding a biologic DMARD or tsDMARD. Specifically, if a patient fails one TNF inhibitor (TNFi)-biologic, options include receiving a second TNFi-biologic versus receiving a DMARD with a different mechanism of action.

The 2018 NICE guideline recommends using various types of DMARDs (other biologic DMARDs, or tsDMARDs) one after another to treat RA patients with active disease despite the use of biologic DMARD, or tsDMARD, without specifying whether the same class/mechanism or a different class/mechanism is preferable.

Key Clinical Points for Biologic Disease-Modifying Antirheumatic Drug–Experienced Patient with Rheumatoid Arthritis

1. In a biologic DMARD–experienced patient with RA with active disease despite the current use of biologic DMARD, the recommendation is to substitute with a DMARD that has a different mechanism of action than the current treatment. In some cases, a medication with the same mechanism of action may also work.
2. If a patient has active RA despite trying one TNFi-biologic, a second TNFi-biologic or a DMARD with a different mechanism of action (non-TNFi or tsDMARD) are options.
3. In a tsDMARD-experienced patient with RA with active disease, the recommendation is to substitute with a medication with a different mechanism of action, that is, a non-TNFi-biologic or a TNFi-biologic (if that had not been tried previously).
4. The higher the number of failed RA DMARD therapies, the more refractory the disease is, and the less likely it is to respond to the current DMARD medication.

TAPERING OF TREATMENT IN PEOPLE WITH RHEUMATOID ARTHRITIS IN LOW DISEASE ACTIVITY OR REMISSION

The 2018 NICE guideline indicates that DMARD dose reduction or a step-down strategy should only be considered after a patient has been in disease remission for at least 1 year without the use of glucocorticoids.

The 2021 ACR guideline indicates the tapering is considered if the patients have been a target of low disease activity or remission for at least 6 months. The 2021 ACR guideline recommended the following in the decreasing rank order for people who are at target for at least 6 months: continuation of all DMARDs at the current dose >> DMARD dose reduction >> DMARD dose reduction and gradual discontinuation >> abrupt DMARD discontinuation. In people with combination DMARD regimens, discontinuation of MTX was recommended over discontinuation of biologic DMARD or tsDMARD.

The 2019 EULAR guideline recommended that if a patient is in persistent remission and has tapered the glucocorticoids to off, then one can consider tapering biologic DMARD or tsDMARD. They recognized that the definition of persistent remission does not exist and may be from 3 to 12 months. Most patients can regain good outcome by the reinstitution of the previous treatment if they flare during the DMARD tapering.

Key Clinical Points for Tapering Disease-Modifying Antirheumatic Drug Therapy in Rheumatoid Arthritis in People Who Achieve Treatment Goal

1. In people who achieve low disease activity or remission, tapering therapy is an option.
2. Most guidelines recommend that patients should be in persistent disease remission when the tapering begins.
3. Tapering of DMARD should be slow, while carefully monitoring for the evidence of active disease.

TREATMENT OF PATIENT WITH RHEUMATOID ARTHRITIS WITH SIGNIFICANT COMORBIDITIES

The 2021 ACR guideline recommended the following to reduce the risk of complications: MTX was recommended over other DMARDs in people with mild and stable parenchymal lung disease, nonalcoholic fatty liver disease, or with subcutaneous nodules; csDMARD over others in people with serious infections; and non-TNFi-biologic or tsDMARD recommended over TNFi-biologic DMARDs in people with heart failure.

The 2019 EULAR and the 2019 NICE guidelines did not make recommendations for people with RA and significant concomitant comorbid conditions. Both guidelines do not address the impact of common comorbidities on the treatment of an RA. However, BSR safety review[26] provides some insights into risks associated with these medications, which can guide treatment in people with other concomitant conditions.

Key Clinical Points for Treating Patient with Rheumatoid Arthritis with Significant Comorbidities

1. Specific DMARD medications may be preferred in patients with RA with comorbidities, to reduce the likelihood of adverse event outcomes.
2. Most guidelines recommend MTX as the preferred DMARD in many of these situations; rituximab is preferred in patients with hypogammaglobulinemia.

RECENT DEVELOPMENTS THAT MAY SIGNIFICANTLY IMPACT THE APPROACH TO RHEUMATOID ARTHRITIS TREATMENT

Recently, the Food and Drug Administration (FDA) made changes to the label of Janus-kinase class of drugs changing the current indication from MTX-experienced to at least one biologic-experienced.[27] This was based on a direct competitor phase IV, FDA-mandated, head-to-head pharmacovigilance study that compared two doses of tofacitinib, a Janus-kinase tsDMARD, with a TNFi-biologic DMARD, either adalimumab or etanercept, in people who failed to respond to MTX and who were 50 years of age or older and had at least one additional cardiovascular risk factor.[28] The study reported lower risks of major adverse cardiovascular event (MACE) and malignancy (excluding nonmelanoma skin cancer) for those treated with TNFi-biologics compared with tofacitinib, both primary end points for the trial. For the two noninferiority coprimary end points, MACE and malignancy, neither noninferiority end point was met; there was a small and numerically (but nonsignificantly) increased risk of MACE and a significantly increased risk for malignancy (excluding nonmelanoma skin cancer) risks with combined tofacitinib arms compared with TNFi-biologic.[28] MACE estimates/100 person-years in ORAL-surveillance were 0.91 for tofacitinib 5 mg twice daily, 1.05 for tofacitinib 10 mg twice daily, and 0.73 for TNFi-biologics. Cancer estimates/100 person-years were 1.13, 1.13 versus 0.77, respectively.[28] Based on the result of this trial,[28] the FDA added a Blackbox warning to the FDA label for all Janus-kinase drugs (tofacitinib, baricitinib, and upadacitinib), and changed the indication from MTX-experienced to biologic-experienced people with RA with active disease.[27]

In my opinion, the label change and the Blackbox warning will impact the current use of tsDMARDs, from previously being used in csDMARD or biologic DMARD-experienced patients with RA with active disease, to now mostly being used in biologic DMARD-experienced patients with RA with active disease. The recent trial provided data only for those who were 50 years or older and had at least one additional cardiovascular risk factor.[28] However, as discussed in the accompanying editorial, these trial results may be getting extrapolated to all age groups, regardless of cardiovascular risk factors.[29]

Although tsDMARDs were options for treatment of patients with active RA despite MTX treatment previously, only the healthiest of such patients who strongly prefer oral treatment may be prescribed tsDMARDs going forward. In most cases, adding biologic DMARDs or other csDMARDs may be preferred. In patients with biologic DMARD failure with active RA, who are old, have a cardiovascular risk factor, or cardiovascular disease, substituting with a biologic with a different mechanism of action is preferred over substituting with a tsDMARD. For others with biologic DMARD failure with active RA, substituting with a biologic DMARD with a different mechanism of action or a tsDMARD is reasonable.

SUMMARY

The first-line treatment of RA is with a csDMARD, such as MTX. For people who continue with moderate-high disease activity despite treatment with therapeutic doses of MTX, data exist for the efficacy of adding a biologic DMARD, another csDMARD, or a tsDMARD. However, the recent Janus-kinase drug label change leaves the addition of a biologic DMARD or another csDMARD as more desired and viable options. Once a biologic DMARD or combination csDMARD have failed to control RA disease activity, substitution with another biologic DMARD or tsDMARD are reasonable options. Future head-to-head trials will help with selection of treatment options for patients with active RA.

CLINICS CARE POINTS

- Use an objective, validated measure of RA disease activity to guide DMARD treatment escalation. Several, validated measaures are available, recommended by the American College of Rheumatology.
- It's best to make treatment decisions after detailed discussions with the patient, considering their values, preferences and risk-benefit views, alongside some attention to the insurance payer restrictions.
- Rapid control of RA disease activity, and sustained low disease activity or remission state in RA is key to optimal quality of life, function and preventing disability in RA.

DISCLOSURE

J.A. Singh has received consultant fees from Schipher, Crealta/Horizon, Medisys, Fidia, PK Med, Two labs Inc, Adept Field Solutions, Clinical Care Options, Clearview Healthcare Partners, Putnam Associates, Focus Forward, Navigant Consulting, Spherix, MedIQ, Jupiter Life Science, UBM LLC, Trio Health, Medscape, WebMD, and Practice Point Communications; and the National Institutes of Health and the American College of Rheumatology. J.A. Singh has received institutional research support from Zimmer Biomet Holdings. J.A. Singh received food and beverage payments from Intuitive Surgical/Philips Electronics North America. J.A. Singh owns stock options in TPT Global Tech, Vaxart Pharmaceuticals, Atyu Biopharma, Adaptimmune Therapeutics, GeoVax Labs, Pieris Pharmaceuticals, Enzolytics Inc, Seres Therapeutics, Tonix Pharmaceuticals Holding Corp, and Charlotte's Web Holdings, Inc. J.A. Singh previously owned stock options in Amarin, Viking, and Moderna Pharmaceuticals. J.A. Singh is on the speaker's bureau of Simply Speaking. J.A. Singh is a member of the executive of Outcomes Measures in Rheumatology, an organization that develops outcome measures in rheumatology and receives arms-length funding from eight companies. J.A. Singh serves on the FDA Arthritis Advisory Committee. J.A. Singh is the chair of the Veterans Affairs Rheumatology Field Advisory Board. J.A. Singh is the editor and the Director of the University of Alabama at Birmingham Cochrane Musculoskeletal Group Satellite Center on Network Meta-analysis. J.A. Singh previously served as a member of the following committees: member, the American College of Rheumatology's (ACR) Annual Meeting Planning Committee and Quality of Care Committees; the Chair of the ACR Meet-the-Professor, Workshop, and Study Group Subcommittee; and the co-chair of the ACR Criteria and Response Criteria subcommittee.

REFERENCES

1. Fraenkel L, Bathon JM, England BR, et al. American College of Rheumatology guideline for the treatment of rheumatoid arthritis. Arthritis Rheumatol 2021; 73(7):1108–23.
2. Smolen JS, Landewé RBM, Bijlsma JWJ, et al. EULAR recommendations for the management of rheumatoid arthritis with synthetic and biological disease-modifying antirheumatic drugs. Ann Rheum Dis 2020;79(6):685–99.
3. Drug treatment for rheumatoid arthritis. 2022. Available at. https://pathways.nice. org.uk/pathways/rheumatoid-arthritis/drug-treatment-for-rheumatoid-arthritis. National Institute for Health and Care Excellence. Accessed March 14, 2022.

4. Bykerk VP, Akhavan P, Hazlewood GS, et al. Canadian Rheumatology Association recommendations for pharmacological management of rheumatoid arthritis with traditional and biologic disease-modifying antirheumatic drugs. J Rheumatol 2012;39(8):1559–82.

5. Smolen JS, Aletaha D, Bijlsma JWJ, et al. Treating rheumatoid arthritis to target: recommendations of an international task force. Ann Rheum Dis 2010;69(4):631–7.

6. Sammaritano LR, Bermas BL, Chakravarty EE, et al. American College of Rheumatology guideline for the management of reproductive health in rheumatic and musculoskeletal diseases. Arthritis Care Res 2020;72(4):461–88.

7. Goodman SM, Springer B, Guyatt G, et al. American College of Rheumatology/American Association of Hip and Knee Surgeons guideline for the perioperative management of antirheumatic medication in patients with rheumatic diseases undergoing elective total hip or total knee arthroplasty. Arthritis Rheumatol 2017;69(8):1538–51.

8. Ledingham J, Gullick N, Irving K, et al. BSR and BHPR guideline for the prescription and monitoring of non-biologic disease-modifying anti-rheumatic drugs. Rheumatology (Oxford) 2017;56(12):2257.

9. Jagpal A, Singh JA. Treatment guidelines in rheumatoid arthritis: optimizing the best of both worlds. Curr Treat Options Rheumatol 2020;6(4):354–69.

10. Mian A, Ibrahim F, Scott DL. A systematic review of guidelines for managing rheumatoid arthritis. BMC Rheumatol 2019;3(1). https://doi.org/10.1186/s41927-019-0090-7.

11. Singh JA, Saag KG, Bridges SL Jr, et al. American College of Rheumatology guideline for the treatment of rheumatoid arthritis. Arthritis Rheumatol 2016;68(1):1–26.

12. Singh JA, Furst DE, Bharat A, et al. 2012 update of the 2008 American College of Rheumatology recommendations for the use of disease-modifying antirheumatic drugs and biologic agents in the treatment of rheumatoid arthritis. Review. Arthritis Care Res (Hoboken) 2012;64(5):625–39.

13. Saag KG, Teng GG, Patkar NM, et al. American College of Rheumatology 2008 recommendations for the use of nonbiologic and biologic disease-modifying antirheumatic drugs in rheumatoid arthritis. Arthritis Rheum 2008;59(6):762–84.

14. Smolen JS, Landewe R, Bijlsma J, et al. EULAR recommendations for the management of rheumatoid arthritis with synthetic and biological disease-modifying antirheumatic drugs: 2016 update. Ann Rheum Dis 2017;76(6):960–77.

15. Smolen JS, Landewe R, Breedveld FC, et al. EULAR recommendations for the management of rheumatoid arthritis with synthetic and biological disease-modifying antirheumatic drugs: 2013 update. Ann Rheum Dis 2014;73(3):492–509.

16. Smolen JS, Landewe R, Breedveld FC, et al. EULAR recommendations for the management of rheumatoid arthritis with synthetic and biological disease-modifying antirheumatic drugs. Ann Rheum Dis 2010;69(6):964–75.

17. Kerschbaumer A, Sepriano A, Smolen JS, et al. Efficacy of pharmacological treatment in rheumatoid arthritis: a systematic literature research informing the 2019 update of the EULAR recommendations for management of rheumatoid arthritis. Ann Rheum Dis 2020;79(6):201.

18. Adalimumab, etanercept, infliximab and abatacept for treating moderate rheumatoid arthritis after conventional DMARDs have failed. Technology appraisal guidance [TA715]. Available at. https://www.nice.org.uk/guidance/ta715. National Institute of Health and Care Excellence (NICE). Accessed March 14, 2022.

19. Adalimumab, etanercept, infliximab, rituximab and abatacept for the treatment of rheumatoid arthritis after the failure of a TNF inhibitor. Technology appraisal guidance [TA195]. Available at. https://www.nice.org.uk/guidance/ta195. National Institute of Health and Care Excellence (NICE). Accessed March 14, 2022.
20. Tofacitinib for moderate to severe rheumatoid arthritis. Technology appraisal guidance [TA480]. Available at. https://www.nice.org.uk/guidance/ta480. National Institute of Health and Care Excellence (NICE). Accessed March 14, 2022.
21. Baricitinib for moderate to severe rheumatoid arthritis. Technology appraisal guidance [TA466]. Available at. https://www.nice.org.uk/guidance/ta466. National Institute of Health and Care Excellence (NICE). Accessed March 14, 2022.
22. Upadacitinib for treating severe rheumatoid arthritis. Technology appraisal guidance [TA665]. Available at. https://www.nice.org.uk/guidance/ta665. National Institute of Health and Care Excellence (NICE). Accessed March 14, 2022.
23. Filgotinib for treating moderate to severe rheumatoid arthritis. Technology appraisal guidance [TA676]. Available at. https://www.nice.org.uk/guidance/ta676. National Institute of Health and Care Excellence (NICE). Accessed March 14, 2022.
24. Rheumatoid arthritis in adults: management. NICE guideline [NG100]. 2022. Available at. https://www.nice.org.uk/guidance/ng100. National Institute of Health and Care Excellence (NICE). Accessed March 14, 2022.
25. Chakravarty K, McDonald H, Pullar T, et al. BSR/BHPR guideline for disease-modifying anti-rheumatic drug (DMARD) therapy in consultation with the British Association of Dermatologists. Rheumatology (Oxford) 2008;47(6):924–5.
26. Holroyd CR, Seth R, Bukhari M, et al. The British Society for Rheumatology biologic DMARD safety guidelines in inflammatory arthritis. Rheumatology (Oxford) 2019;58(2):372.
27. FDA requires warnings about increased risk of serious heart-related events, cancer, blood clots, and death for JAK inhibitors that treat certain chronic inflammatory conditions. Approved uses also being limited to certain patients. 2022. Available at. https://www.fda.gov/drugs/drug-safety-and-availability/fda-requires-warnings-about-increased-risk-serious-heart-related-events-cancer-blood-clots-and-death. U.S. Food and Drug Administration. Accessed February 03, 2022.
28. Ytterberg SR, Bhatt DL, Mikuls TR, et al. Cardiovascular and cancer risk with tofacitinib in rheumatoid arthritis. N Engl J Med 2022;386(4):316–26.
29. Singh JA. Risks and benefits of Janus kinase inhibitors in rheumatoid arthritis: past, present, and future. N Engl J Med 2022;386(4):387–9.

The Meaningful Role of Patients, and Other Stakeholders in Clinical Practice Guideline Development

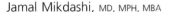

Jamal Mikdashi, MD, MPH, MBA

KEYWORDS

- Clinical guidelines development • Patient stakeholders • Patient partners
- Patient advocacy groups • Role of patients in guidelines development

KEY POINTS

- Patient participation is an integral component in the development of clinical practice guidelines.
- Suboptimal patient engagement signifies a predicament in guideline's legitimacy and transparency.
- Limited budgets, logistic constraints, and discordance in patients' and researchers' perception of a meaningful involvement are some barriers that hinder patient engagement.
- Advancing skill development across various roles within the guideline's process will enrich patient's contribution and allow them to voice their experience, knowledge, perspective, and concerns.
- Continuing patient education and evaluation of their engagement on both outcome and process will facilitate team cohesion, trustworthiness, and value to achieve optimal quality of care.

INTRODUCTION

Clinical practice guidelines (CPGs) are developed to ensure that the treating physician has the exposure to the best evidence-based practices, which is translated into recommendations that are effective in improving patient outcome, preventing morbidity and mortality, and saving resources when providing care.[1] Generated guidelines offer clinical providers with recommendations for decisions frequently faced in clinical practice to promote valuable and desirable outcome but may not adequately convey all uncertainties and nuances of patient care.[2,3]

Division of Rheumatology and Clinical Immunology, University of Maryland School of Medicine, 10 South Pine Street, Suite 834, Baltimore, MD 21201, USA
E-mail address: jmikdash@som.umaryland.edu

Rheum Dis Clin N Am 48 (2022) 691–703
https://doi.org/10.1016/j.rdc.2022.05.002
0889-857X/22/© 2022 Elsevier Inc. All rights reserved.

rheumatic.theclinics.com

Different validated tools and standard methodologies are used including the Grading of Recommendations Assessment, Development, and Evaluation methodology to ensure the methodological rigor and transparency of guidelines development.[4-6] The explicit methods of searching, selection, and grading of the available evidence must safeguard against bias and potential conflict of panelists while incorporating expert input and consensus into the guidelines.[7]

One of the strengths of the CPG process is the consideration of values and preferences of the patients and the engagement of all relevant stakeholders in the development of the CPG recommendations.[8] Patient engagement is hypothesized to increase the likelihood of adoption of the guidelines particularly if the patients are involved in the CPG development build.[9] To strengthen the trust of these recommendations, patient's input must be used at the appropriate questions being asked, the proper outcome being examined, and the patient values and preferences are considered in the interpretation of the evidence and the formulation of the recommendations.[10]

Many recommendations may be based largely on very low-certainty or low certainty evidence; however, consensus statements are easily reached on most statements after prolonged discussions and debate.[11-15] Voting panels would favor strong or conditional recommendation where members of the voting panel agree with the patient panel on the direction and strength of these recommendations. Discordances may occur between patient preferences and physician preferences but these differences reinforce the importance of using a shared decision-making process when dealing with a clinically relevant subject. Nonetheless, at times, it is not possible to represent all patients' viewpoints.

Patient engagement practices in CPG development process represent a continuum. A broad engagement practices process has commonly involved a unidirectional input from patients to investigators via solicitation of viewpoints or experiences to inform guidelines subjects but may be bidirectional information flow and active decision-making and collaborations. Others have advocated for more collaboration than contribution, shared leadership practices, and patient partners embedded as coinvestigators.[16]

The purpose of this article is to discuss the important role of patients and patients' stakeholders in the development of CPG to achieve quality improvement and high value care. Patients are assumed to be a bona fide of the health-care team. Patients' stakeholders in this article are referred to as patients, family members, caregivers, patient partners, patient advocacy groups and members of the public or others to whom the recommendation apply.

This article was developed with the aid of nonsystematic searches of Pub Med and Google Scholar using search terms: "CPGs," "development of practice guidelines," "rheumatic disorders and patient partners," patient advocates, and "role of patients in CPGs."

DEVELOPING GUIDELINES

To optimize patient care, practice guidelines development requires a dialog among the expert practicing physicians, health services researchers, patients, stakeholders, and potential users or evaluators of the guidelines.[17] Specific questions that are related to the scope of the guidelines must be answered by the evidence to justify effectiveness of the recommendations, emphasize gaps in the evidence, and commend a road map to future research.[18]

The method of the CPG development process has evolved over the past 2 decades since the first report by the Institute of Medicine (IOM) on the subject, *Clinical Practice*

Guidelines: Direction for the New Program, emphasizing the optimization of patient care based on building trustworthy guidelines through the involvement of knowledgeable, multidisciplinary panel of experts and representatives from key affected groups, including patients' subgroups.[19,20] Patient involvement is vital for the development of high quality and relevant CPG.

Indeed, the Guidelines International Network (G-I-N), IOM, National Academy of Medicine, National Institute for Health and Care Excellence (NICE), and other research funding and patient organizations have advocated for patients' and other stakeholders' involvement in practice guideline development.[21–24] This is mainly to ensure that the guidelines are relevant to the patients' needs and preferences, which will promote adoption of trustworthy guidelines and increase the adherence to therapeutic strategies, that ultimately improve patient outcome and enhance quality of care and quality of life.

Clinical specialty societies, disease advocacy groups, federally supported Task Forces and other organizations have adopted the current state of CPG developmental process. Societies such as the American College of Rheumatology characterized by long history of CPG development and classification criteria for rheumatic diseases have established developmental procedures and have devoted significant financial resources to craft high-quality guidelines including emphasis on patient's perspective across the guidelines process.[25–31] Other rheumatology organizations have allowed patients to be engaged in the guideline's development process but the number of the patient panels and the degree of patient's involvement varied among different projects and different societies.[32,33]

Nonetheless, the degree of the patients' and other stakeholders' engagement in the CPG development process has expanded overtime. Patient panels are mostly engaged at the deliberation and formulation of the recommendations review and have provided input on their values and preferences, which are discussed and incorporated into the recommendations. Examples of patient panel engagement in the CPG development process is depicted on **Table 1**.

At times, patients are involved in the development of the clinical question Population/Intervention/Comparator/Outcome and have decided on the scope of the guidelines project. A few patients are also engaged in the voting panel where they provide input from the patient perspective and preferences about their personal experience

Table 1
Examples of engagement of patients with rheumatic conditions and other stakeholder in the clinical practice guideline development Process

Year/ Organization	Rheumatic Disease	Patient Panel	Voting Panel	Stakeholders
2018, ACR/NPF	Psoriatic arthritis	9	2	Patient advocates
2021 ACR/VF	GCA, TAK, PAN, GPA	11	2	
2019 ACR/AF	JIA	9 + 2 parents	2	
2017 ACR	GIOP	1	1	
2017 BSR	Gout	2		
2014 SFR	Spondylarthritis	1		Self-help organization
2012 ACR	Gout	1	1	

Abbreviations: ACR, American College of Rheumatology; AF, Arthritis Foundation; BSR, British Society of Rheumatology; GCA, Giant cell arteritis; GPA, granulomatosis polyangiitis; NPF, National Psoriasis Foundation; PAN, polyarteritis nodosa; SFR, French Society of Rheumatology; TAK, Takayasu arteritis; VF, Vasculitis Foundation.

regarding clinical and treatment aspects of their disease and vote on the recommendations. However, patients are not part of the core leadership team, or the literature review team, although patients are engaged at times in the evaluation of the literature review evidence summary.

CHALLENGES IN PATIENT'S ENGAGEMENT IN CLINICAL PRACTICE GUIDELINES DEVELOPMENT PROCESS

Many scientific societies and organizations have increased patient participation in the CPG development during the past several years but their role has been inadequate attributed to limited budgets and logistic constraints (**Box 1**). This is a missed opportunity because guideline without adequate patient participation in the CPG development will reflect poorly on the legitimacy and transparency of the proposed recommendations.[34,35] This is particularly critical when the quality of the evidence base is of low certainty and when there are important tradeoffs between benefit and harms.

Although there are opportunities for patient engagement at each step of the CPG development, challenges exist. Despite educating the patient about guidelines development, a common complaint is the ability of the engaged patients to understand medical terminology and how to participate meaningfully particularly when CPG quality is being assessed.[36] The use of medical jargon and the nature of some of the discussion topics such as ethics applications may make it difficult for patients and other stakeholders to understand and follow what is being discussed.

Although the intent and the relationship building toward meaningful engagement are being applied including the use of nonmedical jargon language, still the feeling of patient tokenism and the empty ritual of participation and not having the real power to affect outcome of discussions limit patient participation.[37] Indeed, the power imbalance between patient participants and the CPG teams of investigators contribute to the feeling of limited utility and value of the patients and other stakeholders' contribution and affect their satisfaction as participants.[38]

Box 1
Reported challenges when engaging patients in the guidelines development process

Lack of clarity on the patient role and objectives

Difficulty understanding medical terminology

Failure to engage patient and other stakeholders on determining guidelines scope

Recruitment difficulties

Inadequate training and support

Uncertainty on how to incorporate patient experience

Discrepancies between the views of patients and physicians

Limited options for patients to voice their views

No willingness to ask questions and communicate needs and workloads

Low stakeholder diversity and power imbalance

Decision-making is not explicit

Lack of trust

Not having full disclosure

Lack of genuine engagement feeling may also arise from inadequate patient team diversity and the absence of patient coleadership and power sharing, and not leaving rooms for discussions or allowing time for authentic partnership.[39] Further, the vague perception of the patients' roles by the patients themselves as well as by the investigators, lack of insight of a clear project expectation, and not allowing adequate time to accommodate patients' disability to accomplish a task are other examples that limit patient participation and time commitment.[40] Patient retention have been limited by the ability to continue to participate in the project due to changes in life circumstances or disease recurrence, emotional tolls, and burnout.

Resources constraints may limit the capability to train and accommodate the needs of the involved patients. Having open conversation with the engaged patients and other stakeholders to identify whether monetary compensation is expected, likelihood of accommodation be offered and what is provided on volunteer basis. Still, the value of patient experience and knowledge, which they contribute depends on the level of the involvement of the patients the skills and expertise they bring forward. Nonetheless, several resources and available guidelines from Canadian Institute of Health Research and Patient Centered Outcomes Research Institute exist about compensation of patients and other stakeholders in health research.[41,42]

Strategies to recruit patients or their representatives, and the extent of patient training, orientation, and methods of engaging patients in the CPG developmental process have varied significantly with each guideline produced and each CPG development group.[43,44] However, the impact of these strategies remains unclear and limits the understanding of what aspects of patient's involvement is likely to be effective.

Patient engagement strategies have been examined by many societies and tool kits have been created; however, it is unclear if these resources are applicable across all contexts of the CPG developmental process.[45] It remains to be determined whether these strategies are applicable across different patient populations with different values or preferences, or those who are vulnerable, older, functionally impaired, or sicker and are often with multimorbidities. Such unique factors may affect patient participation in the CPG development.

Although CPG standard processes acknowledge the incorporation of the patient preferences in the recommendation for good quality, its integration in the CPG development has been inconsistent or in many cases nonexistent.[46,47] Further challenges include the uncertainty of how to encompass the patient illness experience and those with complex clinical syndromes or those with conflict of interest (COI) into the evidence-based guidelines. These challenges may contribute to the discrepancies between the views of the patients and the physician investigators.

The scientific societies must manage COI and disclosure in accordance with their organization policies when developing CPG. COI limitation may not only be applicable to the primary investigators or key members involved in the CPG development process but also include patient panels. Patients and other stakeholders involved in the CPG expert panel and voting panels must be at least greater than 50% free of conflicts. Patient panels should have no financial, intellectual, or personal relationship with parties interested in a particular outcome of their thoughts because that may reduce the trust in the CPG.[48,49]

Many CPG suffered from additional limitations concerning the clinical decision-making process shared between patients and physicians including the timely and effective use of patient-reported outcomes (PROs).[50,51] PROs used in clinical trials have included composite measures that evaluate disease activity, comprehensive assessment of symptoms, physical and mental functional status, and health-related quality of life. Yet, the composite measures of multiple PROs remain suboptimal and problematic to be comprehended by patients and other stakeholders despite their quality of content steered by the Standard Protocol Items: Recommendations for Interventional Trials statement published in 2013.[52]

Many PROs may be regarded by patients as complex and may not reflect important aspects related to the patient needs, values, and preferences such as patient well-being, fatigue, sleep disturbances, and psychological and social aspects of the disease burden. Furthermore, there are few endorsed PRO instruments that are considered by patients as beyond simple measures and lack gold standards. Still, most PRO may cause interpretation difficulties related to patient education, psychosocial diseases, or multimorbidities. Such challenges are more pronounced in patients with rare and complex disorders, patients with multimorbidities and those that are economically disadvantaged.

Effective engagement strategies must be applied at the onset of the project that target adequate patient training or knowledge on factors that may influence patient preferences, or how to generate and report preference-informed guidelines. Resources must focus on continued training of the engaged patients across the CPG development process to achieve a meaningful involvement instead of dependence on surveys, literature reviews, and public comments.

PATIENT VALUES AND PREFERENCES

CPG has been developed with emphasis on patient preferences but embraced no clear method on how patient preferences are identified. The G-I-N PUBLIC Toolkit strategies and AGREE II lists of published literature reviews that stressed the incorporation of patient preference in the CPG development.[10,53] However, several CPG development teams have kept using few patients' panelists, tried to identify preferences through focus groups, and surveys, and many have not reported on how their patient-panelist were engaged or how the patients' informed preferences were established.[54]

To identify and incorporate patient preferences in the CPG development process, CPG leaders must entail formal consultation/interviews of participated patients who can provide meaningful preferences and do approve of reviewed published literature that is provided in lay language for medical terms. Nonetheless, limited data exists regarding best practices (**Box 2**) on "how" to obtain patients' views or whether single strategies are sufficient.[55]

Ascertaining patient views and preference requires careful attention to the dynamic interaction of interpersonal, biological, psychological, and socio-environmental contexts that influence the well-being and the health of the patients.[56,57] Patient preferences relate to the patient's perceptions, views, values, and objectives for their health and their lives, and to the manner that the patients use on contemplating the prospect of benefit, harms, costs, inconveniences when dealing with interventional and therapeutic options.

Decision-making based on the patient preference must be simple to comprehend, and each outcome related to management options must be addressed to help patient participants with their selection of the alternative therapies. Informed patients may choose not to follow the proposed CPG if it does not encompass their own preferences and do not appeal to their emotional and social influences.

Further, the timing to solicit patient preferences remains a challenge. To facilitate patient engagement early in the CPG development, the timing should at least be during the formulation of the clinical question and the knowledge synthesis.[58] Indeed, patients are engaged in the CPG development during knowledge synthesis,

Box 2 **Best practices in engaging patients in the guideline's development**
Adequate stakeholder diversity
Involvement of patients and other stakeholders from inception of the process
Patient partnership and coleadership
Equal voices of patients and investigators
Patients' influence on topic priorities and guidelines relevance and quality
Proper patient education and preparation
Define roles, responsibilities, and expectations
Adequate training tailored to patients needs
Patient involvement in rapid reviews
Strong team communication and positive feedback
Balanced and manageable workload
Building trust, satisfaction, sense of accomplishment, and gained valuable experience
Creating longitudinal relationship with patients and investigators

recommendation development, draft revision, and at the creation of lay-targeted guidelines material. Nonetheless, patient engagement is rarely performed at the onset of the CPG development for subject decision-making, outlining the scope of the project or during the review process by the panelist committees.

Attention is required on who should be invited to ascertain patient preferences. Systemic methods must be applied on who are the patient stakeholders be it the patients, patient partners, patient advocates, general publics, or those patients who recently faced the challenges with decision related to the scope of the CPG.[59] Direct patient education with long-term patient commitment, and counseling on how to provide input and how to balance different patient preference perspective may be helpful. However, lack of time, funds, and patient's knowledge encumber incorporation of patient preferences or may lead to loss of interest by invited patients and other stakeholders, and devalue their input, and ultimately offer poor-quality contemporary guidelines.

Systematic assessment of the patient engagement in the CPG development must have the same thoroughness and iterative approach such as the guidelines team members and expert panels responsible for the guideline's formulation. Incorporating patients' preferences require the involvement of diverse patient population, who have different illnesses experience attributed to cultural, ethnic, and religious backgrounds with different languages and geographic regions.

FRAMEWORK FOR ENHANCING CLINICAL PRACTICE GUIDELINES THROUGH CONTINUOUS PATIENT ENGAGEMENT ALONG THE ENTIRE CLINICAL PRACTICE GUIDELINES DEVELOPMENT PROCESS

Patients should be recognized as experts with important contribution that have the capability to inform health-care policy makers about their patients' valued outcomes, needs, and views. The leadership of the CPG team requires different preparation to empower all team members (researchers, patients, other stakeholders from the start of the guidelines process to help in the design, carryout, and management of the guideline's projects. To advocate for patients' views and achieve a meaningful engagement of patients and other stakeholders, different strategies may be placed at each step of the entire CPG development process including direct patient engagement.

Several proposed frameworks for the steps to engage patients and other stakeholders are published and are typically performed at the developer or committee levels.[60,61] Formal consultation with patients to determine the priority topics is underscored as ascertained by AGREE II instrument.[62] Active solicitation of guidelines topic through websites allowing the public to submit topic nomination or through electronic mails, community meetings and focus groups or contacting advocacy groups are more successful steps likely to engage patients. Engaging patients in prioritizing topic nominations or the selected topics can ensure that the guidelines developers are addressing patient's needs. Despite limited resources, guidelines developer must promote the needs of the patients and their selection of the prioritized topics.

Engagement of the patients early in the decision process is critical once the guidelines topic is chosen. Framing the guidelines questions and developing research plan to their best advantage is meaningful to the patients involved. Patient input can help determine the important patient's preferences, outcome selection, patient's harms, as well as the targeted population of interest that may benefit from the guidelines. Direct patient involvement in the early stages of CPG development process will help in the posting of the guidelines plans for public comments as advocated by the United States Preventive Services Task Force and NICE.[16]

Training is required should patients and other stakeholders need to be engaged in the completion of the systemic reviews. NICE identifies the training needed to achieve the ability to understand scientific articles as part of the minimum skills set for patients and caregivers.[63] Other organization such as Consumers United for Evidence-based Healthcare can offer participants with training on evidence-based medicine and critical assessment of the evidence.[64] Patient representatives may as well post drafts of evidence summaries and conclusion for the public comments, which may improve guidelines awareness and implementation.

In addition to the endorsement of the recommendations and participation in the dissemination of the CPG, patient engagement must continue if there is a public reason for the topic reconsideration and whether and when the guidelines require updates apart from new evidence.

Continued evaluation of the patients' roles and responsibilities across the recommendation development process provide insights into the preferences and views of the patients and ensure that the recommendations facilitate the patients' needs and outcomes. Metrics need to be identified that evaluate success and quality of patient partnership as well as satisfaction of the patient engagement experience. Patients must determine whether their contribution was meaningful, effective, and how to improve their future participation.

SUMMARY

CPG development from idea conception to policy making requires a demanding duty from our medical profession. Patient engagement in CPG development process represents an opportunity to leverage not only the patients' selective values and preferences but the knowledge of the patient needs, skills and experiences that lead to improve patient clinical outcome. A meaningful patient involvement must foster a culture change that emphasizes patient and other stakeholders' engagement at each step of the entire CPG development process.

Strategies must address barriers that affect patient engagement and pursue resolutions to challenges such as limited resources availability that facilitate substantial partnership with patients and other stakeholders and accommodate patient's disability, scheduling adjustment, and personal needs. Attention to disease-specific states of mild, moderate, or severe disease activity and patient-reported burden of functional disability or cognitively impairment must be contemplated in the CPG development process. Implementation of effective patient engagement strategies across CPG development process must be incorporated to mitigate unbalanced power dynamics and meet the purpose of the CPG to deliver the best practices and clinical decision support needed to improve patient-relevant outcome and enhance the CPG's validity, trustworthiness, and rigor.

CLINICS CARE POINTS

- Patient engagement at each step of the clinical practice guidlines process is paramount to acheive trustworthiness and value in the proposed guidleines to achieve optimal quality of care.
- A meaningful patients and other stakeholders involvement must incorporate patient needs, experience, values, preferences, and presence of disability and multimorbidities.
- Innovative strategies require better understanding of opportunities, challaneges and future directions in patient and other stakeholders engagement in the guidelines developemental process.

DISCLOSURE

The author has nothing to disclose.

REFERENCES

1. Field MJ, Lohr KN, editors. Clinical practice guidelines: directions for a new program. Institute of Medicine. Washington (DC): National Academic Press; 1990.
2. Shekelle PG, Woolf SH, Eccles M, et al. Developing guidelines. BMJ 1999;31: 593–6.
3. Yao X, Xia J, Yinghui J, et al. Methodological approaches for developing, reporting, and assessing evidence-based clinical practice guidelines: A systematic survey. J Clin Epidemiol 2022;146:77–85.
4. Zhang Y, Akl EA, Schünemann HJ. Using systematic reviews in guideline development: the GRADE approach. Res Synth Methods 2019;10:312–29.
5. The AGREE Collaboration. Appraisal of Guidelines for Research & Evaluation AGREE) Instrument. Available at: http://www.agreecollaboration.org/.
6. Banno M, Tsujimoto Y, Kataoka Y. The majority of reporting guidelines are not developed with the Delphi method: a systematic review of reporting guidelines. J Clin Epidemiol 2020;124:50–7.
7. Page MJ, McKenzie JE, Higgins JP. Tools for assessing risk of reporting biases in studies and syntheses of studies: a systematic review. BMJ open 2018;8: e019703.
8. Montori VM, Brito JP, Murad MH. The optimal practice of evidence-based medicine: Incorporating patient preferences in practice guidelines. JAMA 2013;310: 2503–4.
9. Kim C, Berta WB, Gagliardi AR. Exploring approaches to identify, incorporate and report patient preferences in clinical guidelines: qualitative interviews with guideline developers. Patient Educ Couns 2021;104:703–8.

10. Eccles MP, Grimshaw JM, Shekelle P, et al. Developing clinical practice guidelines: target audiences, identifying topics for guidelines, guideline group composition and functioning and conflicts of interest. Implement Sci 2012;7:1–8.

11. Mikuls TR, Johnson SR, Fraenkel L, et al. American College of rheumatology guidance for the management of rheumatic disease in adult patients during the COVID-19 pandemic: version 1. Arthritis Rheumatol 2020;72:1241–51.

12. Mikuls TR, Johnson SR, Fraenkel L, et al. American College of Rheumatology Guidance for the management of rheumatic disease in adult patients during the COVID-19 Pandemic: version 2. Arthritis Rheumatol 2020;72:e1–2.

13. Hersh A, Yazdany J. Clinical practice guidelines and diagnostic uncertainty in the management of early rheumatoid arthritis. J Rheumatol 2009;36:863–4.

14. Onel KB, Horton DB, Lovell DJ, et al. 2021 American College of Rheumatology Guideline for the Treatment of Juvenile Idiopathic Arthritis: Recommendations for Nonpharmacologic Therapies, Medication Monitoring, Immunizations, and Imaging. Arthritis Rheumatol 2022;74:570–85.

15. Curtis JR, Johnson SR, Anthony DD, et al. American college of rheumatology guidance for COVID-19 vaccination in patients with rheumatic and musculoskeletal diseases: version 4. Arthritis Rheumatol 2022;74:e21–36.

16. Armstrong MJ, Gronseth GS, Gagliardi AR, et al. Participation and consultation engagement strategies have complementary roles: A case study of patient and public involvement in clinical practice guideline development. Health Expect 2020;23:423–32.

17. Altman RD, Schemitsch E, Bedi A. Assessment of clinical practice guideline methodology for the treatment of knee osteoarthritis with intra-articular hyaluronic acid. Semin Arthritis Rheum 2015;45:132–9.

18. Lantos PM, Rumbaugh J, Bockenstedt LK, et al. Clinical practice guidelines by the Infectious Diseases Society of America (IDSA), American Academy of Neurology (AAN), and American College of Rheumatology (ACR): 2020 guidelines for the prevention, diagnosis and treatment of Lyme disease. Clin Infect Dis 2021;72:e1–48.

19. Kung J, Miller RR, Mackowiak PA. Failure of clinical practice guidelines to meet institute of medicine standards: two more decades of little, if any, progress. Arch Int Med 2012;172:1628–33.

20. Goodman RA, Boyd C, Tinetti ME, et al. IOM and DHHS meeting on making clinical practice guidelines appropriate for patients with multiple chronic conditions. Ann Fam Med 2014;12:256–9.

21. Qaseem A, Forland F, Macbeth F, et al. Board of Trustees of the Guidelines International Network. Guidelines International Network: toward international standards for clinical practice guidelines. Ann Int Med 2012;156:525–31.

22. de Wit MP, Berlo SE, Aanerud GJ, et al. European League Against Rheumatism recommendations for the inclusion of patient representatives in scientific projects. Ann Rheum Dis 2011;70:722–6.

23. Goodman SM, Miller AS, Turgunbaev M, et al. Clinical practice guidelines: incorporating input from a patient panel. Arthritis Care Res 2017;69:1125–30.

24. National Institute for Health and Clinical Excellence. The guidelines manual. London: National Institute for Health and Clinical Excellence; 2007. Available at: www.nice.org.uk.

25. Hahn BH, Mcmahon MA, Wilkinson A, et al. American College of Rheumatology guidelines for screening, treatment, and management of lupus nephritis. Arthritis Care Res 2012;64:797–808.

26. Khanna D, Khanna PP, Fitzgerald JD, et al. 2012 American College of Rheumatology guidelines for management of gout. Part 2: therapy and antiinflammatory prophylaxis of acute gouty arthritis. Arthritis Care Res 2012;64:1447–61.

27. Buckley L, Guyatt G, Fink HA, et al. 2017 American College of Rheumatology guideline for the prevention and treatment of glucocorticoid-Induced osteoporosis. Arthritis Rheumatol 2017;69:1521–37.

28. Ringold S, Angeles-Han ST, Beukelman T, et al. 2019 American College of Rheumatology/Arthritis Foundation guideline for the treatment of juvenile idiopathic arthritis: therapeutic approaches for non-systemic polyarthritis, sacroiliitis, and enthesitis. Arthritis Care Res 2019;71:717–34.

29. Singh JA, Guyatt G, Ogdie A, et al. 2018 American College of Rheumatology/National Psoriasis Foundation guideline for the treatment of psoriatic arthritis. Arthritis Rheumatol 2019;71:5–32.

30. Kolasinski SL, Neogi T, Hochberg MC, et al. 2019 American College of Rheumatology/Arthritis Foundation guideline for the management of osteoarthritis of the hand, hip, and knee. Arthritis Rheumatol 2020;72:220–33.

31. Maz M, Chung SA, Abril A, et al. 2021 American College of Rheumatology/Vasculitis Foundation guideline for the management of giant cell arteritis and Takayasu arteritis. Arthritis Care Res 2021;73:1071–87.

32. Wendling D, Lukas C, Paccou J, et al. Recommendations of the French Society for Rheumatology (SFR) on the everyday management of patients with spondyloarthritis. Joint Bone Spine 2014;81:6–14.

33. Hui M, Carr A, Cameron S, et al. The British Society for Rheumatology guideline for the management of gout. Rheumatology 2017;56:e1–20.

34. Woolf SH, Grol R, Hutchinson A, et al. Potential benefits, limitations, and harms of clinical guidelines. BMJ 1999;318:527–30.

35. Boivin A, Green J, van der Meulen J, et al. Why consider patients' preferences: A discourse analysis of clinical practice guideline developers. Med Care 2009;908–15.

36. van Wersch A, Eccles M. Involvement of consumers in the development of evidence based clinical guidelines: practical experiences from the North of England evidence based guideline development programme. BMJ Qual Saf 2001; 10:10–6.

37. Hahn DL, Hoffmann AE, Felzien M, et al. Tokenism in patient engagement. Fam Pract 2017;34:290–5.

38. Boden C, Edmonds AM, Porter T, et al. Patient partners' perspectives of meaningful engagement in synthesis reviews: A patient-oriented rapid review. Health Expect 2021;24:1056–71.

39. Tricoci P, Allen JM, Kramer JM, et al. Scientific evidence underlying the ACC/AHA clinical practice guidelines. JAMA 2009;301:831–41.

40. Burns KK, Bellows M, Eigenseher C, et al. 'Practical' resources to support patient and family engagement in healthcare decisions: a scoping review. BMC Health Serv Res 2014;14:1–5.

41. Canadian Institutes of Health Research. Considerations when paying patient partners in research. 2019. Available at: http://cihr-irsc.gc.ca/e/51466.html.

42. Patient Centered Outcomes Research Institute. Financial compensation of patients, caregivers, and patient/caregiver organizations engaged in PCORI-funded research as engaged research partners. 2015. Available at: https://www.pcori.org/sites/default/files/PCORI-Compensation-Framework-for-Engaged-Research-Partners.pdf.

43. Armstrong MJ, Mullins CD, Gronseth GS, et al. Recommendations for patient engagement in guideline development panels: a qualitative focus group study of guideline-naive patients. PLoS One 2017;12:e0174329.

44. Morin SN, Djekic-Ivankovic M, Funnell L, et al. Patient engagement in clinical guidelines development: input from> 1000 members of the Canadian osteoporosis patient network. Osteoporos Int 2020;31:867–74.

45. Carman KL, Dardess P, Maurer M, et al. Patient and family engagement: a framework for understanding the elements and developing interventions and policies. Health Aff 2013;32:223–31.

46. Hochberg MC, Altman RD, April KT, et al. American College of Rheumatology 2012 recommendations for the use of nonpharmacologic and pharmacologic therapies in osteoarthritis of the hand, hip, and knee. Arthritis Care Res 2012; 64:465–74.

47. Constantin T, Foeldvari I, Anton J, et al. Consensus-based recommendations for the management of uveitis associated with juvenile idiopathic arthritis: the SHARE initiative. Ann Rheum Dis 2018;77:1107–17.

48. Schünemann HJ, Wiercioch W, Etxeandia I, et al. Guidelines 2.0: systematic development of a comprehensive checklist for a successful guideline enterprise. CMAJ 2014;186:E123–42.

49. Nejstgaard CH, Bero L, Hróbjartsson A, et al. Conflicts of interest in clinical guidelines, advisory committee reports, opinion pieces, and narrative reviews: associations with recommendations. Cochrane Database Syst Rev 2020;12(12): MR000040.

50. Fautrel B, Alten R, Kirkham B, et al. Call for action: how to improve use of patient-reported outcomes to guide clinical decision making in rheumatoid arthritis. Rheumatol Int 2018;38:935–47.

51. Toupin-April K, Barton JL, Fraenkel L, et al. OMERACT Development of a Core Domain Set of Outcomes for Shared Decision-making Interventions. J Rheumatol 2019;46:1409–14.

52. Chan AW, Tetzlaff JM, Altman DG, et al. SPIRIT 2013 statement: defining standard protocol items for clinical trials. Ann Int Med 2013;158:200–7.

53. Institute of Medicine of the National Academies. In: Eden J, Wheatley B, McNeil B, et al, editors. Knowing what Works in health care. A Roadmap for the nation. Washington, DC: National Academies Press; 2008.

54. Blackwood J, Armstrong MJ, Schaefer C, et al. How do guideline developers identify, incorporate and report patient preferences? An international cross-sectional survey. BMC Health Serv Res 2020;20:458.

55. Kim C, Armstrong MJ, Berta WB, et al. How to identify, incorporate and report patient preferences in clinical guidelines: A scoping review. Health Expect 2020;23: 1028–36.

56. Epstein RM, Peters E. Beyond information: exploring patients' preferences. JAMA 2009;302:195–7.

57. Hsiao B, Fraenkel L. Patient preferences for rheumatoid arthritis treatment. Curr Opin Rheumatol 2019;31:256–63.

58. van Overbeeke E, Janssens R, Whichello C, et al. Design, Conduct, and Use of Patient Preference Studies in the Medical Product Life Cycle: A Multi-Method Study. Front Pharmacol 2019;10:1395.

59. van Overbeeke E, Vanbinst I, Jimenez-Moreno AC, et al. Patient Centricity in Patient Preference Studies: The Patient Perspective. Front Med (Lausanne) 2020; 7:93.

60. Armstrong MJ, Rueda JD, Gronseth GS, et al. Framework for enhancing clinical practice guidelines through continuous patient engagement. Health Expect 2017; 1:3–10.
61. Armstrong C, Grant S, Kinnett K, et al. Participant experiences with a new online modified-Delphi approach for engaging patients and caregivers in developing clinical guidelines. Eur J Pers Cent Healthc 2019;7:476.
62. Duarte-García A, Cavalcante M, Arabelovic S, et al. Systematic appraisal of the American College of Rheumatology clinical practice guidelines. ACR Open Rheumatol 2019;1:188–93.
63. Petkovic J, Riddle A, Akl EA, et al. Protocol for the development of guidance for stakeholder engagement in health and healthcare guideline development and implementation. Syst Rev 2020;9:b21.
64. Han G, Mayer M, Canner J, et al. Development, implementation and evaluation of an online course on evidence-based healthcare for consumers. BMC Health Serv Res 2020;20:928.

Treatment Guidelines in Vasculitis

Tanaz A. Kermani, MD, MS[a], Kenneth J. Warrington, MD[b], Anisha B. Dua, MD, MPH[c],*

KEYWORDS

- Vasculitis • Giant cell arteritis • Takayasu arteritis • Polyarteritis nodosa
- Granulomatosis with polyangiitis • Microscopic polyangiitis
- Eosinophilic granulomatosis with polyangiitis • Treatment Guidelines

KEY POINTS

- The American College of Rheumatology/Vasculitis Foundation guidelines aim to provide advice on diagnostic/evaluation strategies, therapeutic options, and long-term management of these complex diseases based on the best available evidence to date.
- The diagnosis of vasculitis often requires a combination of clinical, serologic, radiographic, and pathologic evaluation.
- There are differences in recommendations across rheumatologic societies due to variability in available diagnostic modalities and access to and cost of therapeutics.
- Specific biomarkers for the diagnosis and monitoring of vasculitis and availability of safe, targeted therapeutics are needed and ongoing areas of active research in vasculitis.

GIANT CELL ARTERITIS

Introduction

Giant cell arteritis (GCA) is a granulomatous large-vessel vasculitis that involves the cranial arteries, the aorta and its proximal branches.[1] It clinically affects the elderly population with ischemic complications including vision loss, stroke, and limb claudication. The treatment of GCA has historically relied heavily on long-term glucocorticoids (GC), with resultant adverse effects, toxicities, as well as frequent relapses. A better understanding of the pathophysiology of GCA has led to the development of GC-sparing therapies, whereas advances in imaging have allowed insight into the prevalence and implications of extracranial large-vessel involvement.

[a] University of California Los Angeles, 2020 Santa Monica Boulevard, Suite 540, Santa Monica, CA 90404, USA; [b] Mayo Clinic, 200 First Street Northwest, Rochester, MN 55905, USA; [c] Northwestern University Feinberg School of Medicine, 675 North St. Clair Street, Suite 14-100, Chicago, IL 60611, USA
* Corresponding author.
E-mail address: Anisha.dua@northwestern.edu

Rheum Dis Clin N Am 48 (2022) 705–724
https://doi.org/10.1016/j.rdc.2022.03.006
0889-857X/22/© 2022 Elsevier Inc. All rights reserved.

rheumatic.theclinics.com

Discussion

Overview

The American College of Rheumatology/Vasculitis Foundation (ACR/VF) Guideline included 7 recommendations on diagnostic testing and 15 on medical management, surgical intervention, and disease monitoring[2,3] (**Table 1**). Ungraded position statements were made by the voting panel when there was not enough evidence to support a graded recommendation but the question addressed a commonly encountered clinical question, thus guidance was provided based on general views of the voting panel. There were 2 ungraded position statements, and all recommendations were conditional except 1 strong recommendation to clinically monitor patients long-term who are in clinical remission. The European Alliance of Associations of Rheumatology (EULAR) has also published recommendations on the diagnosis and management of GCA[4] (**Table 2**).

Diagnostic evaluation

Early diagnosis and initiation of treatment in GCA is critical to improve outcomes. The ACR/VF guideline recommends obtaining a temporal artery biopsy over a temporal artery ultrasound in patients suspected of having GCA.[2,3] Further recommendations include obtaining a unilateral biopsy of at least 1 cm within 2 weeks of initiating GC therapy. However, EULAR recommends an early imaging test with ultrasound of the temporal ± axillary arteries as the first imaging modality in patients with suspected predominantly cranial GCA.[5] Much of this discrepancy centers on expertise in ultrasound for diagnosing GCA. Ultrasound is a noninvasive, inexpensive, and accessible test that can be used to assess various arteries affected by GCA. However, ultrasound is highly user-dependent, and features, such as the halo sign, tend to resolve soon after GC exposure. In one study, the sensitivity of ultrasound decreased following the use of GC, from 92% after 0 to 1 days, to 80% after 2 to 4 days, to 50% after more than 4 days of GC[6]. There has been interest and research in incorporating ultrasound into fast-track clinics to develop and validate algorithmic approaches that might help risk stratify patients and allow for low-probability patients to avoid undergoing further testing and unnecessary medications.[7–9] Although ultrasound demonstrates utility in the diagnostic algorithm including the ability to assess some extracranial vessels, pathologic diagnosis may have utility in prognostication, and histologic features remain positive for a longer period of time in patients exposed to GC. In one study, repeat temporal artery biopsy remained positive in 70% of patients at 3 months after GC exposure and in 44% of patients at 12 months.[10] To date, an ideal radiographic, serologic, or pathologic biomarker that can consistently and accurately diagnose, detect relapses, and risk-stratify patients in need of specific types of immunomodulating therapy in GCA has remained elusive.

The ACR/VF guideline recommends large-vessel imaging in all suspected and confirmed cases of GCA, whereas EULAR recommendations note that noninvasive imaging may be helpful to support the diagnosis of large-vessel involvement in GCA but do not specifically recommend it in all suspected cases.[2,3,5] The optimal modality and frequency of noninvasive imaging for monitoring patients with GCA has not been established and likely should reflect baseline large-vessel involvement along with their clinical course.

Glucocorticoids

One of the most feared complications of GCA is vision loss and early initiation of GC once diagnosis is suspected is important in the prevention of vision loss.[11,12] In patients with threatened vision loss, the ACR/VF guideline recommends intravenous

Table 1
Summary of recommendations from the American College of Rheumatology/Vasculitis foundation guideline

	GCA	TAK	PAN	GPA/MPA	EGPA
Diagnosis	Temporal artery biopsy, noninvasive large-vessel imaging	No specific recommendations	Deep-skin biopsy, nerve and muscle biopsy, abdominal vascular imaging	No specific recommendations	No specific recommendations but echocardiogram in all patients at diagnosis
Glucocorticoid (GC) use	High dose oral GC, IV GC for cranial ischemia Duration guided by patient's condition, values, and preferences	High-dose oral GC, IV GC for severe disease, organ-threatening ischemia and if needed for pediatric patients Taper to 0 mg after 6–12 mo	High-dose oral GC, IV GC for life-threatening or organ-threatening disease	IV GC or high-dose oral GC Reduced-dose GC regimen for taper Duration guided by patient's condition, values, and preferences	IV GC or high-dose oral GC Duration guided by patient's condition, values, and preferences
Remission induction (severe disease)	High-dose GC and tocilizumab	High-dose GC and AZA or MTX or TNFi	High-dose GCA and cyclophosphamide	High-dose GC and RTX No plasma exchange	High-dose GC and RTX or cyclophosphamide
Remission maintenance	Tocilizumab	AZA or MTX or TNFi	Immunosuppressive agent (other than CYC)	Fixed-dose RTX	AZA or MTX or MMF
Monitoring	Clinical evaluation, acute phase reactants Long-term clinical monitoring	Clinical evaluation, acute phase reactants, large-vessel imaging Long-term clinical monitoring	Abdominal vascular imaging	No specific recommendations	No specific recommendations
Management of specific disease phenotype/subset	Not applicable	Not applicable	TNFi for patients with DADA2	MTX for induction in nonsevere GPA/MPA	Mepolizumab for patients with nonsevere disease

Abbreviations: DADA2, Deficiency of adenosine deaminase 2; EGPA, eosinophilic granulomatosis with polyangiitis; GC, glucocorticoids; GCA, giant cell arteritis; GPA, granulomatosis with polyangiitis; IV, intravenous; MPA, microscopic polyangiitis; MTX, methotrexate; PAN, polyarteritis nodosa; RTX, rituximab; TAK, Takayasu arteritis; TNFi, tumor necrosis factor inhibitor.

Table 2
Comparison of American college of rheumatology/vasculitis foundation guideline and European alliance of associations of rheumatology recommendations for the management of large-vessel vasculitis[2–4]

	GCA		TAK	
	ACR/VF	**EULAR**	**ACR/VF**	**EULAR**
Diagnosis	Temporal artery biopsy Noninvasive large-vessel imaging in ALL suspected and newly diagnosed GCA	Temporal artery ultrasound ± axillary arteries Noninvasive large-vessel imaging to support a diagnosis of large-vessel GCA	No recommendations	Referral to a tertiary care center if possible for diagnosis and confirmation with large-vessel imaging
GC use	IV pulse GCs in cranial ischemia High-dose oral GC in GCA without cranial ischemia	Same Same	High-dose GC, IV pulse in severe disease	High-dose GC, no comment about IV use
Adjunctive therapy	In newly diagnosed GCA, use oral GC + TCZ	Use adjunctive TCZ or MTX only in select patients (relapsing, refractory, high risk of GC side effects)	MTX, AZA or TNFi in all patients with active disease	Adjunctive immunosuppression with MTX, AZA, leflunomide or MMF in all patients with active disease
Biologic therapy			TNFi favored over tocilizumab. TNFi can be used as first line adjunctive therapy	If fail immunosuppressive therapy with DMARD, either TNFi or tocilizumab may be used

Abbreviations: ACR/VF, American College of Rheumatology/Vasculitis Foundation; DMARD, disease modifying antirheumatic drug; EULAR, European alliance of associations of rheumatology; GC, glucocorticoids; GCA, giant cell arteritis; IV, intravenous; MMF, mycophenolate mofetil; MTX, methotrexate; TAK, takayasu arteritis; TNFi, tumor necrosis factor inhibitor.

(IV) pulse GC,[2,3] although this is based on very-low level evidence from conflicting retrospective studies.[2,3] Given the concern for progressive vision loss in this at-risk population, IV GC are used in clinical practice for patients who present with signs of cranial ischemia. In line with this ACR/VF guideline, EULAR also recommends using 0.25 to 1g IV methylprednisolone daily for up to 3 days in GCA patients with acute visual loss or amaurosis fugax.[4]

In patients with newly diagnosed GCA without cranial ischemic symptoms, recommendations are to initiate high-dose GC (over moderate or pulse dose GC).[2,3] This is in keeping with EULAR recommendations to use 40 to 60 mg/d of GC for the induction of remission.[4] The trial of tocilizumab (TCZ) in GCA (GiACTA) demonstrated that we have historically been using more GCs than necessary.[13] Although GCs are still central in our management of GCA, strategies to limit their use while still optimizing the health of our GCA patients have been discovered.

Controversies: the role of tocilizumab

Because of the significant toxicities associated with high-dose, long-term GC exposure, multiple other therapeutics have been evaluated for their GC-sparing effect. The ACR/VF guideline recommends the use of oral GC with TCZ over oral GC alone for patients with newly diagnosed GCA.[2,3]

Although the efficacy of TCZ has clearly been demonstrated in GCA, the questions of cost, allocation, and whether there is a subset of patients that would benefit most from this initial treatment remains controversial. Between 30% and 60% of patients do not relapse on GC monotherapy and are able to taper to less than 5 mg/d at 1 year.[14-17] EULAR recommends the treatment with GC monotherapy with adjunctive therapy such as TCZ reserved for select patients who have refractory or relapsing disease, or for those at increased risk of GC-related adverse effects or complications.[4,18]

EULAR recommendations also include methotrexate (MTX) as an alternative and less costly, GC-sparing agent. Data around the efficacy of MTX in patients with GCA has been debated with clinical trials providing conflicting results.[19-21] The METOGiA trial (NTC03892785) will compare weekly TCZ to 0.3 mg/kg/wk of MTX over 1 year to evaluate the efficacy and cost-effectiveness of these 2 agents in GCA.

Questions remain regarding the optimal length of TCZ treatment. Long-term data show that less than 50% of patients with GCA who discontinued TCZ after 1 year had sustained remission during the next 2 years, with most patients suffering from relapse.[22] Furthermore, there were no clear clinical, biomarker, or imaging features that reliably predicted GCA patients at higher risk of relapse.

Summary

The ACR/VF guideline supports the use of temporal artery biopsy for the initial diagnosis of GCA, which is in contrast to EULAR recommendations to use temporal artery ultrasound. Although both societies endorse large-vessel imaging, the indications for and frequency of imaging remains unclear. TCZ has been demonstrated to allow for GC reduction and is recommended by the ACR/VF along with GC at diagnosis for patients with GCA, whereas EULAR recommends TCZ or MTX in relapsing and resistant cases. This discordance likely reflects the limited availability and high cost of TCZ. Fortunately, multiple other medications/biologics are being tested in phase 2 and 3 clinical trials in GCA, so the landscape will continue to change.

TAKAYASU ARTERITIS
Introduction

Takayasu arteritis (TAK) is a granulomatous large-vessel vasculitis predominantly affecting the aorta and/or its major branches.[1] The revised International Chapel Hill Consensus Conference suggests using age of less than 50 years to distinguish TAK from GCA.[1] The estimated incidence is 1.11 per million person years with an estimated prevalence ranging from 8.4 per million in the United States to 40 per million in Japan.[23] Vascular inflammation in TAK leads to vascular damage with arterial stenosis, occlusion, or dilatation.[24]

Discussion

Overview
The ACR/VF guideline for TAK included 20 recommendations (19 conditional, 1 strong) and 1 ungraded position statement.[2,3] For all of the recommendations, the level of evidence available was rated as low or very low. The only strong recommendation was to monitor patients over time. EULAR has also published recommendations on the management of large-vessel vasculitis.[4,5]

Diagnostic evaluation
The ACR/VF guideline includes no statements about diagnostic modalities for TAK.[2,3] EULAR recommends confirmation of large-vessel vasculitis with imaging modalities and referral to a center with expertise for diagnosis of TAK.[4] Computed tomography (CT), magnetic resonance imaging (MRI), and positron emission tomography (PET) supersede conventional angiography given their ability to assess the vessel wall for signs of inflammation, and, the lumen.[25] EULAR recommends MRI as the modality of choice to diagnose TAK, with PET, CT, or ultrasound as alternatives, with the caveat that ultrasound cannot assess the thoracic aorta.[5]

Glucocorticoids
The ACR/VF guideline recommends the treatment with high-dose GC over IV GC for both newly diagnosed and relapsing active, severe disease.[2,3] They recommend consideration of IV GC for those with the most severe disease, recognizing that there is no evidence supporting use of IV GC over oral GC.[2,3] Despite the absence of well-designed clinical trials, pulse steroids are often used to treat severe manifestations in rheumatic diseases given anti-inflammatory effects on a wide range of immune cells via genomic mechanisms.[26] IV steroids were also considered for children if needed for compliance or to reduce adverse effects on growth.[2,3] EULAR also recommends initiation of high-dose GC for the induction of remission in TAK without any statement about pulse steroids.[4] As opposed to EULAR recommendations to taper GC to a target dose of 10 mg or less after 1 year, the ACR/VF recommends tapering off GC for patients in remission after 6 to 12 months of therapy.[2,3]

Controversies: adjunctive therapy and the role of biologics
It is increasingly recognized that most patients with TAK have relapsing disease.[24] Both EULAR and the ACR/VF recommend initiation of additional immunosuppressive therapy at diagnosis over treatment with GC alone.[2–4] The data for GC-sparing medications in TAK is based on retrospective and open label studies, and therefore, the choice is based on patient-specific factors including plans for childbearing, comorbidities, and adverse effect profile. As opposed to EULAR recommendations to start with conventional immunosuppressive therapy and add biologic therapy in cases of refractory disease, the ACR/VF guideline considers tumor necrosis factor inhibitors (TNFi) as first line along with conventional immunosuppressive therapy.[2–4] This difference may

reflect other factors including cost and access to biologic therapies. The recommendations on choice of biologic therapy also differ. EULAR recommends TNFi or TCZ for refractory disease, whereas based on currently available data, ACR/VF favors TNFi over TCZ in TAK.[2–4] Although TCZ was studied in a randomized phase III clinical trial, the study only included 36 patients and the primary endpoint of time to first relapse was no different between those treated with TCZ or placebo, although there was some steroid-sparing effect of TCZ.[27]

Surgical management

ACR/VF guideline recommends medical management over surgical intervention in nearly all cases including worsening ischemia (except coronary involvement or impending/progressive tissue or organ infarction), persistent limb claudication, renovascular hypertension, cranial/cervical disease (without symptoms or multi-vessel involvement).[2,3] Both EULAR recommendations and the ACR/VF guideline recommend deferring intervention in patients with active disease when possible with ACR/VF also including a statement recommending the use of high-dose GC in those with active disease perioperatively.[2–4] Neither provides any guidance on preference of surgical treatment versus noninvasive vascular interventions in patients with TAK, and EULAR recommends a multidisciplinary team approach.[2–4]

Controversies: the role of imaging in disease activity assessment

Despite their limitations, the use of acute phase reactants is recommended along with clinical assessment to evaluate disease activity in the EULAR recommendations and the ACR/VF guideline.[2–4] In patients who are in clinical remission but with elevated markers of inflammation, ACR/VF recommends observation.[2,3]

Most experts agree imaging is an important in the care of patients with TAK.[28] ACR/VF guideline recommends routine noninvasive imaging in TAK.[2,3] In contrast, EULAR does not recommend routine imaging for disease activity assessment in patients in clinical and biochemical remission but in cases of suspected relapse, or, to monitor structural damage.[2–5]

The significance of imaging findings such as vessel wall edema and enhancement remain unclear and debated.[29–31] A controversial recommendation of the ACR/VF guideline is the escalation of therapy in cases of clinical remission with signs of inflammation on imaging including edema or enhancement in a new vascular territory.[2,3] Although experts would agree a new area of stenosis warrants escalation of therapy, there is no clear evidence that vessel wall edema or enhancement, even in a new area, represents active inflammation or risk for progression/development of new vascular damage.[2,3] The guideline acknowledges this uncertainty and recommends the imaging findings be reviewed with a radiologist before making any treatment decisions.[24]

Summary

The ACR/VF guideline provides helpful recommendations for the medical and surgical management of TAK. Areas of uncertainty include the best imaging modalities for diagnosis and monitoring. Furthermore, the significance of findings such as vessel wall edema or enhancement and whether they represent disease activity or vessel remodeling are unknown. The role of TCZ for the treatment of TAK needs to be further investigated. There remains a need for therapeutics that better control the inflammation and reduce risk of relapses and damage over time.

POLYARTERITIS NODOSA

Introduction

Polyarteritis nodosa (PAN) is a rare, systemic necrotizing vasculitis that predominantly involves medium-sized and small arteries without involvement of arterioles, venules, or capillaries.[1] Generally, antineutrophil cytoplasmic antibodies (ANCA) are absent. The incidence of PAN is about 1 to 8 per million population, and the estimated prevalence is 31 per million; this form of vasculitis occurs mainly between the age of 40 and 60 years and is more common in men.[23] PAN can be broadly divided into primary (idiopathic) and secondary (related to Hepatitis B virus [HBV] infection) forms. Deficiency of adenosine deaminase 2 (DADA2) has overlapping clinical features with PAN; this monogenic form of vasculitis which is caused by mutations in the ADA2 gene generally presents in childhood but may also manifest in young adults.[32]

Discussion

Overview

The 2021 ACR/VF guideline included 16 recommendations and 1 ungraded position statement for the evaluation and treatment of patients with the systemic, idiopathic form of PAN[33,34] (**Table 3**). The guideline addresses neither the management of patients with cutaneous PAN nor the management of patients with HBV-related PAN.[33,34] In contrast, the older EULAR recommendations review treatment of both idiopathic PAN as well as HBV-related PAN, noting that antiviral therapy is an essential component of the treatment strategy for the latter condition.[35] It should be emphasized that most of the ACR/VF recommendations for PAN are conditional due to the lack of consistent high-quality evidence in this field.

Diagnostic evaluation

PAN should be included in the differential diagnosis of patients with a systemic, inflammatory multisystem illness and progressive end organ dysfunction. The diagnosis of PAN may be delayed due to the rare nature of disease, the often nonspecific initial patient symptoms, and the necessity to exclude vasculitis mimics particularly infection. Unfortunately, specific diagnostic biomarkers are not available for PAN, although the presence of elevated inflammatory markers may be a useful clue to the diagnosis. Therefore, imaging studies and tissue biopsy constitute essential components of the diagnostic evaluation.[33,34] The ACR/VF guideline emphasizes the use of abdominal vascular imaging for the diagnosis of PAN, recognizing that CT angiography, magnetic resonance angiography, and catheter-direct angiography are all reasonable diagnostic modalities, with the latter providing greatest resolution and sensitivity.[33,34] Characteristic findings on conventional angiography such as multiple microaneurysms of the hepatic, mesenteric, and renal artery branches are often diagnostic of PAN. Depending on the pattern of clinical involvement, muscle, nerve, or deep-skin biopsies for histopathologic confirmation of medium vessel vasculitis may be required. The characteristic histologic findings may be missed in a superficial "punch" skin biopsy; therefore, ACR/VF guidelines specify that a deep biopsy ("double" punch or excisional) is preferable based on expert opinion.[33,34] Although not specifically addressed in the ACR/VF recommendations, it is generally advisable that patients with suspected PAN should be evaluated and subsequently managed at (or in close collaboration with) centers that have expertise in vasculitis, as noted in the EULAR guidelines.[35]

Treatment recommendations

Once a diagnosis of PAN is established, and mimics have been reasonably excluded, the clinician should assess the degree of disease severity to tailor treatment

Table 3
Comparison of American College of Rheumatology/Vasculitis Foundation Guideline and European Alliance of Associations of Rheumatology Recommendations for Management of Polyarteritis nodosa[33–35]

	ACR/VF	EULAR
Diagnosis	Abdominal vascular imaging Deep-skin biopsy Nerve and muscle biopsy	Biopsy confirmation of vasculitis is recommended; site not specified in guideline
GC use	IV GC initially	High-dose GC
Remission induction	CYC and high-dose GC	Same
Plasmapheresis	Not recommended	Recommended for patients with HBV-related PAN
Remission maintenance	Immunosuppressive agent (other than CYC)	Same

Abbreviations: ACR/VF, American College of Rheumatology/Vasculitis Foundation; CYC, cyclophosphamide; EULAR, European alliance of associations of rheumatology; GC, glucocorticoids; HBV, hepatitis B virus; IV, intravenous; PAN, polyarteritis nodosa.

accordingly. Severe disease with life-threatening or organ-threatening manifestations (eg, renal disease, mononeuritis multiplex, mesenteric ischemia, coronary involvement, limb/digit ischemia) should be treated with GC combined with cyclophosphamide (CYC) to induce disease remission.[36] The use of initial IV GC can be considered for patients with urgent need to limit end organ damage, although this is based on very-low level of evidence and most patients can be treated with high-dose oral GC.[33,34,36] This treatment strategy outlined in the ACR/VF guidelines is consistent with the EULAR recommendations for the management of medium vessel vasculitis.[33–35]

Treatment with CYC is typically continued for 3 to 6 months (adjusted for renal and hematologic parameters), after which it is replaced with a remission maintenance agent such as MTX or azathioprine (AZA), for total treatment duration of about 18 months—a strategy that is based on expert opinion and extrapolation of data from clinical trials of other forms of vasculitis. The ACR/VF guidelines discourage the use of rituximab (RTX) over CYC and recommend against the use of plasma exchange for the treatment of PAN due to the lack of evidence supporting these treatment modalities.[33,34] Patients with intolerance to CYC and those with nonsevere disease manifestations should be treated with immunosuppressive agents such as MTX or AZA (in combination with GC).[33,34] It is worth noting that the ACR/VF guideline does not support treating patients with PAN with GC monotherapy due to risk of toxicity, although there is some evidence to support this strategy for patients with limited disease. Given the lack of clinical trial data evaluating the optimal duration of GC treatment in PAN, the ACR/VF guideline committee did not provide specific recommendations on when to discontinue GC; they suggested individualized therapy and shared decision-making incorporating patient preferences.[33,34] The treatment of refractory vasculitis is particularly challenging, and the ACR/VF guideline addresses this by recommending that if a patient is on immunosuppressive therapy with MTX or AZA and has ongoing active disease, then treatment should be escalated to use of CYC.[33,34] Although this is entirely appropriate, clinicians should also remain vigilant for other conditions for example, infection that can mimic "refractory vasculitis" and may need an entirely different approach to management.[33–35]

The only strong recommendation in the ACR/VF guideline pertains to the management of patients with DADA2. Based on clinical experience, patients with DADA2 seem to respond remarkably well to the treatment with TNFi resulting in reduction in the risk of stroke.[37] Given the apparent difference in treatment response between idiopathic PAN and DADA2, clinicians should consider testing for DADA2 when younger patients with medium vessel vasculitis have atypical PAN manifestations such as stroke.

Summary

The recent ACR/VF guideline provides clinicians with a framework for the evaluation and treatment of patients with systemic idiopathic PAN. The diagnostic evaluation for PAN hinges on vascular imaging and tissue biopsy as specific biomarkers are lacking. Treatment is directed at abrogating the systemic inflammatory process to limit end organ damage; GC and CYC are the mainstay of therapy for remission induction in severe disease. Maintenance of remission is generally achieved with a conventional immunosuppressive agent, and optimal duration of treatment remains unclear. Several unmet needs remain in the management of PAN, including the availability of targeted and safer therapeutic agents.

GRANULOMATOSIS WITH POLYANGIITIS AND MICROSCOPIC POLYANGIITIS
Introduction

Granulomatosis with polyangiitis (GPA) and microscopic polyangiitis (MPA) are ANCA-associated vasculitides (AAV) that cause necrotizing inflammation of the small-sized and medium-sized blood vessels. These two disease entities have many overlapping clinical manifestations and management considerations; thus, they have been studied together in randomized clinical trials and were addressed simultaneously in the ACR/VF guideline.[38,39]

Discussion

Overview

Twenty-six conditional recommendations and 5 ungraded position statements were developed to guide the management of MPA/GPA.[38,39] All of them had very low to moderate levels of supporting evidence. Most recommendations address remission induction and remission maintenance in severe and nonsevere disease. EULAR/the European Renal Association-European Dialysis and Transplant Association (ERA-EDTA) have also developed guidelines for the management of AAV[40] (**Table 4**).

Glucocorticoids

A major advancement in the management of AAV has been seen with our ability to use less GCs than ever before. Recent trials have demonstrated that we can use significantly less GCs without compromising clinical efficacy and with improvements in quality of life measures. A large randomized trial in patients with severe MPA and GPA showed that a reduced dose GC arm was as effective as the standard GC arm in regards to end-stage renal disease or death, with fewer serious infections, and more than 50% less GC exposure at 3 months.[41] The ACR/VF recommends a reduced-dose GC regimen over a standard regimen for remission induction in severe disease.[38,39] Since the literature review for the guidelines, 2 other important trials have evaluated the role of lower dose GCs in AAV. These trials reinforced the importance of and the noninferiority of a lower dose GC regimen as well as the ability of avacopan, an oral C5a inhibitor, to reduce GC burden in severe MPA/GPA.[42,43]

Controversies: rituximab or cyclophosphamide for remission induction in severe disease

In severe, active GPA/MPA, the ACR/VF guidelines recommend induction of remission using RTX over CYC in addition to high-dose GCs.[38,39] In contrast, EULAR/ERA-EDTA recommends either CYC or RTX for the induction of remission.[40,44] RTX was shown to be noninferior to CYC in a pivotal clinical trial but this trial excluded patients on mechanical ventilation or with a creatinine level of more than 4 mg/dL.[45] The clinical trial that evaluated RTX in newly diagnosed AAV with severe renal manifestations was confounded by additional use of IV CYC as part of the induction regimen.[46] Various factors can influence the choice of induction therapy including patient comorbidities, childbearing plans, infectious risks, MPO or PR3 positivity, new or relapsing disease, as well as cost and availability. Access to RTX in the United States, comparable efficacy, and favorable side effect profile, led to the ACR/VF recommendation of RTX over CYC for induction in severe disease.[38,39]

Importantly, in refractory disease, both ACR/VF guideline and EULAR/ERA-EDTA recommend switching to the alternative agent (RTX→CYC or CYC→RTX).[38–40] The ACR/VF also recommends that severe relapses in patients not on RTX for maintenance therapy should be reinduced with RTX but those who are on RTX for maintenance therapy should be induced with CYC.[38,39] The timing of the relapse in relation to RTX, the maintenance regimen being used, patient comorbidities, and clinical history should all be incorporated into the decision-making process in individual cases.[38,39]

Clinical controversies: the role of plasmapheresis

Another area of controversy in the induction of remission is the role of plasmapheresis in those with severe renal involvement and/or alveolar hemorrhage. The ACR/VF guideline recommends against adding plasmapheresis for the induction of remission in active glomerulonephritis or diffuse alveolar hemorrhage.[38,39] The MEPEX trial required a serum creatinine level of greater than 5.8 mg/dl for entry and showed that plasmapheresis decreased the risk of end-stage renal disease but did not decrease mortality.[47] The more recent PEXIVAS trial demonstrated that there was no benefit to adding plasmapheresis to standard induction therapy (with CYC/RTX and GCs) in terms of progression to end-stage renal disease or mortality (28% plasmapheresis vs 31% no plasmapheresis, $P = .27$).[41] These results informed the ACR/VF recommendation against plasmapheresis in severe GPA and MPA.[38,39] Interestingly, a meta-analysis including both of these trials showed a decreased risk of end-stage renal disease with plasmapheresis (HR 0.27; 95% CI 0.53–0.98).[48] EULAR/ERA-EDTA recommendations, published before the PEXIVAS trial, recommend plasmapheresis for AAV patients with severe renal failure (creatinine >500 mmol/L, 5.7 mg/dL) and state that it be should be considered in those with other life-threatening manifestations of disease, such as diffuse alveolar hemorrhage.[40] Although the ACR/VF guideline recommends using RTX for induction and no plasmapheresis in cases of severe renal and/or pulmonary involvement, a patient's specific clinical scenario will undoubtedly inform therapeutic decision-making.[38,39]

Treatment of nonorgan or life-threatening disease

In nonsevere GPA/MPA, the ACR/VF recommends induction with a combination of GCs and MTX over using RTX, CYC, AZA, mycophenolate mofetil (MMF), trimethoprim/sulfamethoxazole, or GCs alone.[38,39] EULAR/ERA-EDTA recommends induction with a combination of GCs with either MTX or MMF for induction in nonorgan threatening disease.[40]

Table 4
Comparison of American College of Rheumatology/Vasculitis Foundation Guideline and European Alliance of Associations of Rheumatology/European Renal Association- European Dialysis and Transplant Association Recommendations for Management of Anti-neutrophil cytoplasmic antibody-associated vasculitis[38–40]

	GPA/MPA		EGPA	
	ACR/VF	EULAR/ERA-EDTA	ACR/VF	EULAR/ERA-EDTA
Diagnosis	No specific recommendations	Biopsy to establish diagnosis	No specific recommendations apart from echocardiogram in all patients	Biopsy to establish diagnosis
GC use	Reduced-dose GC regimen	Target prednisone dose between 7.5 and 10 mg daily after 3 mo of treatment	High-dose GC, duration guided by patient's condition, values, and preferences	High dose GC, goal 7.5–10 mg by month 3, continuation of low-dose GC for remission maintenance
Remission induction	High-dose or pulse GC + RTX in severe disease	GC + RTX or CYC in severe disease	High-dose GC and RTX or CYC	Same
Plasmapheresis	Do not use	Consider in glomerulonephritis and severe diffuse alveolar hemorrhage	No specific comment for EGPA (guidelines as for GPA/MPA)	Same
Remission maintenance	RTX Duration of GC and non-GC therapy guided by patients' clinical condition, preferences, and values	Low-dose GC + AZA, RTX, MTX, or MMF Continue for 24 mo following induction of sustained remission	AZA or MTX or MMF Duration of GC use guided by patient's condition, values, and preferences No comment about duration of therapy	Same Low-dose GC continued Duration therapy 24 mo

Abbreviations: ACR/VF, American College of Rheumatology/Vasculitis; AZA, azathioprine; CYC, cyclophosphamide; EGPA, eosinophilic granulomatosis with polyangiitis; EULAR/ERA-EDTA, European Alliance of Associations of Rheumatology/European Renal Association- European Dialysis and Transplant Association; GC, glucocorticoids; GPA, granulomatosis with polyangiitis; MMF, mycophenolate mofetil; MPA, microscopic polyangiitis; MTX, methotrexate; RTX, rituximab.

Remission maintenance

Once remission is induced with either CYC or RTX, the ACR/VF recommends the use of RTX for maintenance therapy.[38,39] Second-line options for maintenance therapy are AZA or MTX, with third-line options including MMF or leflunomide. A trial using RTX 500 mg IV on day 0, 14, then q 6 months compared with AZA, after induction with IV CYC, showed superiority of RTX with fewer major relapses and improved quality of life measures.[49] When AZA was compared with MTX after CYC induction, there was no significant difference in relapse rates or serious adverse events.[50] We do not have comparative trials for specific dosing and timing of RTX for maintenance but based on available data, the dose ranges between 500 and 1000 mg of IV RTX every 4 to 6 months.[51,52] The ACR/VF recommendations are to use scheduled or fixed dosing RTX rather than dosing based on CD19 B cell count or ANCA titers.[38,39] EULAR/ERA-EDTA recommendations for remission maintenance support using a combination of low-dose GCs and either AZA, RTX, MTX, or MMF and continuing therapy for at least 24 months following induction of sustained remission.[40] The length of maintenance therapy is not specifically detailed in the ACR/VF guideline and providers should consider patient factors such as infections, medication tolerance, disease phenotype, history of relapses, and risk for further relapses.

Summary

The ACR/VF guidelines recommend RTX over CYC for the induction of remission in severe MPA/GPA and recommend against plasmapheresis. This is in contrast to EULAR/ERA-EDTA recommendations that support the use of either CYC or RTX for the induction of remission as well as plasmapheresis in cases of glomerulonephritis or diffuse alveolar hemorrhage. Trials have increasingly demonstrated that we are able to effectively induce remission with less GC exposure in our patients with MPA/GPA. Maintenance therapy with fixed-dose RTX should be used, although the length of optimal treatment is unclear. In nonsevere disease, the ACR recommends treatment with MTX for remission induction.

EOSINOPHILIC GRANULOMATOSIS WITH POLYANGIITIS

Introduction

Eosinophilic granulomatosis with polyangiitis (EGPA, previously Churg-Strauss) is a small-vessel vasculitis characterized by eosinophil-rich and necrotizing granulomatous inflammation often involving the respiratory tract with features including asthma and peripheral eosinophilia along with vasculitic manifestations.[1,53] It is the rarest of the 3 forms of AAV with an estimated incidence of 0.14 to 4.0 per million and estimated prevalence up to 32.9 per million.[23] As opposed to GPA and MPA, ANCA is frequently absent (55%–65% negative).[53]

Discussion

Overview

The ACR/VF guideline for EGPA included 15 conditional recommendations and 5 ungraded position statements.[38,39] For all of the recommendations, the level of evidence available was rated as low or very low. The guideline also addressed the use of immunosuppression to treat vasculitic manifestations of EGPA but did not specifically address asthmatic and allergic manifestations of EGPA. EULAR/ERA-EDTA recommendations for treatment of AAV do not separate management of EGPA from GPA/MPA.[40]

Glucocorticoids

Both statements relating to GC use in the ACR/VF guideline for EGPA were ungraded position statements. The first recommendation is for IV pulse GC or high-dose oral GC for active severe diseases.[38,39] The only other statement related to GC use is that the duration of therapy be guided by the patient's clinical condition, values, and preferences. EULAR/ERA-EDTA recommendations for the management of AAV include high-dose GC (1 mg/kg/d) for the induction of remission in EGPA with taper to 7.5 to 10 mg/d by month 3.[40] They recommend continuation of low-dose GC for remission-maintenance.[40]

Controversies: rituximab, cyclophosphamide, or mepolizumab for remission induction

Clinical trials in EGPA are scarce with the treatment based on data from other forms of AAV. For remission induction, the ACR/VF guideline also appropriately considers the severity of disease manifestations.

Despite long-standing experience with CYC and limited data for RTX, ACR/VF guideline includes an ungraded position statement recommending CYC or RTX for remission induction in patients with active, severe EGPA.[38,39] They cite the absence of comparative effectiveness of CYC and RTX as the basis for this recommendation. They did provide scenarios where one drug might be preferred over another including CYC in patients with active cardiac involvement, whereas RTX may be favored in patients with positive ANCA, glomerulonephritis, prior CYC use, or those at risk for gonadal toxicity from CYC.[38,39] A recent systematic review of currently available observational studies for RTX in EGPA found that 80% of patients treated with RTX achieved complete or partial remission with higher response in the p-ANCA-positive subgroup but the high degree of heterogeneity limited applicability to clinical practice.[54] The Rituximab in Eosinophilic Granulomatosis with Polyangiitis (REOVAS) trial (NTC02807103) is a phase III randomized controlled trial comparing CYC versus RTX in EGPA and should provide much needed data on this important question. EULAR/ERA-EDTA recommendations also include CYC or RTX for remission induction for EGPA but although 88% of the panel agreed with use of CYC, only 59% agreed with use of RTX.[40]

The ACR/VF guideline also conditionally recommends CYC or RTX over mepolizumab in patients with active, severe EPGA.[38,39] This is appropriate because patients with active, severe disease were excluded from the clinical trial evaluating mepolizumab in EGPA.[55]

In patients with active but nonsevere disease, the ACR/VF guideline has several conditional recommendations.[38,39] Overall, treatment with mepolizumab and GC was generally favored for this patient population.[38,39] However, GC along with adjunctive immunosuppressive therapy such as AZA, MTX, or MMF was preferred to GC monotherapy, whereas the use of CYC or RTX was discouraged.[38,39] For nonorgan threatening disease, EULAR/ERA-EDTA recommends treatment with GC and MTX or MMF.[40] There are no statements regarding the use of mepolizumab in the EULAR/ERA-EDTA recommendations because the recommendations were published before the results of the trial were available.[40,55]

Remission maintenance

The ACR/VF guideline conditionally recommends treatment with MTX, AZA, or MMF for remission maintenance in patients who received induction therapy with CYC, extrapolating from studies in other forms of AAV.[38,39] These therapies were favored over mepolizumab given paucity of data for mepolizumab in this subset of patients. RTX was not recommended for remission maintenance given lack of data but was suggested if it was used as induction therapy or in cases where there were contrain-dications to the other options.[38,39] No recommendations are made about duration of therapy.[38,39] EULAR/ERA-EDTA recommendations include AZA, MTX, MMF, or RTX for remission maintenance (only data for AZA available for EGPA) with continuation of therapy for 2 years.[40]

Treatment of relapses

The ACR/VF guideline includes 5 conditional recommendations on the treatment of re-lapses.[38,39] In patients who relapse with severe manifestations after an initial response to the treatment with CYC, they recommend switching to RTX over retreating with CYC based on data from an observational study of RTX in relapsing/refractory EGPA.[38,39] Cardiac involvement is listed as an exception again where retreatment with CYC may be considered. In patients with initial response to RTX who relapse with severe manifestations, retreatment with RTX is suggested over switching to CYC.[38,39] They recommend using mepolizumab to treat a nonsevere relapse occur-ring in patients on immunosuppressive therapy, as supported by the clinical trial of mepolizumab in EGPA.[38,39,55] Mepolizumab is also favored over adjunctive immuno-suppressive therapy in patients on GC monotherapy who have a relapse, and, over omalizumab including in patients with elevated IgE.[38,39] For relapsing disease, EULAR/ERA-EDTA recommend using the same algorithm as new disease with GC and retreatment with CYC or RTX to induce remission.[40]

Summary

It is clear that EGPA is different from the other forms of AAV. Whether there are subsets within EGPA with the ANCA-positive subtype more closely resembling MPA/GPA re-mains unclear. As opposed to GPA/MPA, the role of CYC or RTX for remission induc-tion needs to be elucidated. The role of mepolizumab as adjunctive therapy in patients with severe manifestations also needs further study.

Clinics Care Points

- Temporal artery biopsy of at least 1 cm on the affected side is the preferred method for confirming a diagnosis of giant cell arteritis (GCA).
- Large-vessel involvement is underrecognized and screening with noninvasive imaging should be pursued in patients with suspected/newly diagnosed GCA.
- In newly diagnosed GCA with threatened vision loss, pulse IV glucocorticoids (GC) should be used.
- Newly diagnosed GCA patients should be induced with glucocorticoids plus to-cilizumab (TCZ), though the optimal length of TCZ treatment has not been defined.

Clinics Care Points

- The diagnosis of Takayasu arteritis (TAK) should be confirmed by large-vessel imaging.
- Patients with active TAK should be treated with high-dose GC and started on adjunctive immunosuppressive therapy.
- TNFi is currently preferred over the use of TCZ.
- Longitudinal follow-up should include clinical assessment, measurement of acute phase reactants and large-vessel imaging.

Clinics Care Points

- Patients with suspected polyarteritis nodosa (PAN) should be evaluated with abdominal vascular imaging.

- Patients with suspected PAN may require tissue biopsy for confirmation of the diagnosis; the optimal site for biopsy depends on specific vasculitic manifestations.
- Severe, idiopathic PAN should be treated with GC and cyclophosphamide (CYC) for 3 to 6 months before transitioning to less intense immunosuppressive therapy.

Clinics Care Points

- Patients with new onset severe granulomatosis with polyangiitis (GPA)/microscopic polyangiitis (MPA) should be induced with rituximab (RTX) over CYC along with a rapid GC taper.
- Once remission is achieved, scheduled RTX dosing should be used for maintenance, although the length of treatment is unclear.
- In refractory disease, RTX should be switched to CYC or vice-versa.
- In severe relapsing disease, RTX should be used for induction unless the patient is on RTX maintenance therapy, in which case, CYC should be used.
- In nonsevere GPA/MPA, methotrexate (MTX) along with GCs should be used for the induction of remission.

Clinics Care Points

- The treatment of eosinophilic granulomatosis with polyangiitis (EGPA) is based on the severity of the disease and organs affected.
- The decision regarding CYC or RTX for remission induction should be made considering several factors including organs affected, ANCA positivity, patient preferences (eg, desire to preserve fertility), and currently available data.
- Adjunctive immunosuppressive therapy in addition to GC is recommended in most cases.
- Mepolizumab plays a role in the management of nonsevere manifestations and relapsing disease but further studies are needed regarding its utility in patients with severe disease.

SUMMARY

The recent ACR/VF guideline provides a useful framework for the evaluation and treatment of patients with systemic vasculitis. Most of the recommendations were conditional given absence of strong data for many important clinical questions. Diagnostic modalities such as imaging studies are important for large-vessel vasculitis and PAN, whereas tissue biopsy for diagnosis is important for GCA, PAN, and AAV. Common themes include the use of GC with adjunctive therapy for remission induction. With more effective GC-sparing therapies, strategies evaluating shorter GC exposure to minimize adverse effects are becoming increasingly important. Duration of therapy remains unclear for many of these conditions, and the decision is often individualized based on the severity of disease and damage, clinical course including relapses, and patient preferences. All patients with vasculitis warrant long-term follow-up to evaluate for relapses but also complications of the disease and its treatment.

DISCLOSURE

Dr T.A. Kermani has nothing to disclose. Dr K.J. Warrington has received clinical trial support from Kiniksa and Eli Lilly & Co; honoraria from Chemocentryx. Dr A.B. Dua has received honoraria from Chemocentryx, Novartis, and Abbvie.

REFERENCES

1. Jennette JC. Overview of the 2012 revised International Chapel Hill Consensus Conference nomenclature of vasculitides. Clin Exp Nephrol 2013;17:603–6.
2. Maz M, Chung SA, Abril A, et al. 2021 american college of rheumatology/vasculitis foundation guideline for the management of giant cell arteritis and takayasu arteritis. Arthritis Rheumatol 2021;73:1349–65.
3. Maz M, Chung SA, Abril A, et al. 2021 American College of Rheumatology/Vasculitis Foundation Guideline for the Management of Giant Cell Arteritis and Takayasu Arteritis. Arthritis Care Res (Hoboken) 2021;73:1071–87.
4. Hellmich B, Agueda A, Monti S, et al. 2018 Update of the EULAR recommendations for the management of large vessel vasculitis. Ann Rheum Dis 2020;79:19–30.
5. Dejaco C, Ramiro S, Duftner C, et al. EULAR recommendations for the use of imaging in large vessel vasculitis in clinical practice. Ann Rheum Dis 2018;77:636–43.
6. Hauenstein C, Reinhard M, Geiger J, et al. Effects of early corticosteroid treatment on magnetic resonance imaging and ultrasonography findings in giant cell arteritis. Rheumatology (Oxford) 2012;51:1999–2003.
7. Monti S, Bartoletti A, Bellis E, et al. Fast-Track Ultrasound Clinic for the Diagnosis of Giant Cell Arteritis Changes the Prognosis of the Disease but Not the Risk of Future Relapse. Front Med (Lausanne) 2020;7:589794.
8. Oshinsky C, Bays AM, Sacksen I, et al. Vascular ultrasound for giant cell arteritis: establishing a protocol using vascular sonographers in a fast-track clinic in the United States. ACR Open Rheumatol 2022;4(1):13–8.
9. Sebastian A, Tomelleri A, Kayani A, et al. Probability-based algorithm using ultrasound and additional tests for suspected GCA in a fast-track clinic. RMD Open 2020;6(3):e001297.
10. Maleszewski JJ, Younge BR, Fritzlen JT, et al. Clinical and pathological evolution of giant cell arteritis: a prospective study of follow-up temporal artery biopsies in 40 treated patients. Mod Pathol 2017;30:788–96.
11. Gonzalez-Gay MA, Blanco R, Rodriguez-Valverde V, et al. Permanent visual loss and cerebrovascular accidents in giant cell arteritis: predictors and response to treatment. Arthritis Rheum 1998;41:1497–504.
12. Hayreh SS, Zimmerman B, Kardon RH. Visual improvement with corticosteroid therapy in giant cell arteritis. Report of a large study and review of literature. Acta Ophthalmol Scand 2002;80:355–67.
13. Stone JH, Tuckwell K, Dimonaco S, et al. Trial of Tocilizumab in Giant-Cell Arteritis. N Engl J Med 2017;377:317–28.
14. Alba MA, Garcia-Martinez A, Prieto-Gonzalez S, et al. Relapses in patients with giant cell arteritis: prevalence, characteristics, and associated clinical findings in a longitudinally followed cohort of 106 patients. Medicine (Baltimore) 2014;93:194–201.
15. Labarca C, Koster MJ, Crowson CS, et al. Predictors of relapse and treatment outcomes in biopsy-proven giant cell arteritis: a retrospective cohort study. Rheumatology (Oxford) 2016;55:347–56.
16. Martinez-Lado L, Calvino-Diaz C, Pineiro A, et al. Relapses and recurrences in giant cell arteritis: a population-based study of patients with biopsy-proven disease from northwestern Spain. Medicine (Baltimore) 2011;90:186–93.

17. Stone JH, Tuckwell K, Dimonaco S, et al. Glucocorticoid Dosages and Acute-Phase Reactant Levels at Giant Cell Arteritis Flare in a Randomized Trial of Tocilizumab. Arthritis Rheumatol 2019;71:1329–38.

18. Mackie SL, Dejaco C, Appenzeller S, et al. British Society for Rheumatology guideline on diagnosis and treatment of giant cell arteritis. Rheumatology (Oxford) 2020;59:e1–23.

19. Hoffman GS, Cid MC, Hellmann DB, et al. A multicenter, randomized, double-blind, placebo-controlled trial of adjuvant methotrexate treatment for giant cell arteritis. Arthritis Rheum 2002;46:1309–18.

20. Spiera RF, Mitnick HJ, Kupersmith M, et al. A prospective, double-blind, randomized, placebo controlled trial of methotrexate in the treatment of giant cell arteritis (GCA). Clin Exp Rheumatol 2001;19:495–501.

21. Jover JA, Hernandez-Garcia C, Morado IC, et al. Combined treatment of giant-cell arteritis with methotrexate and prednisone. a randomized, double-blind, placebo-controlled trial. Ann Intern Med 2001;134:106–14.

22. Adler S, Reichenbach S, Gloor A, et al. Risk of relapse after discontinuation of tocilizumab therapy in giant cell arteritis. Rheumatology (Oxford) 2019;58:1639–43.

23. Watts RA, Hatemi G, Burns JC, et al. Global epidemiology of vasculitis. Nat Rev Rheumatol 2022;18:22–34.

24. Tombetti E, Mason JC. Takayasu arteritis: advanced understanding is leading to new horizons. Rheumatology (Oxford) 2019;58:206–19.

25. Schafer VS, Jin L, Schmidt WA. Imaging for Diagnosis, Monitoring, and Outcome Prediction of Large Vessel Vasculitides. Curr Rheumatol Rep 2020;22:76.

26. Strehl C, Ehlers L, Gaber T, et al. Glucocorticoids-All-Rounders Tackling the Versatile Players of the Immune System. Front Immunol 2019;10:1744.

27. Nakaoka Y, Isobe M, Takei S, et al. Efficacy and safety of tocilizumab in patients with refractory Takayasu arteritis: results from a randomised, double-blind, placebo-controlled, phase 3 trial in Japan (the TAKT study). Ann Rheum Dis 2018; 77:348–54.

28. Aydin SZ, Direskeneli H, Merkel PA. International Delphi on Disease Activity Assessment in Large-vessel V. Assessment of Disease Activity in Large-vessel Vasculitis: Results of an International Delphi Exercise. J Rheumatol 2017;44: 1928–32.

29. Kato Y, Terashima M, Ohigashi H, et al. Vessel Wall Inflammation of Takayasu Arteritis Detected by Contrast-Enhanced Magnetic Resonance Imaging: Association with Disease Distribution and Activity. PLoS One 2015;10:e0145855.

30. Quinn KA, Ahlman MA, Malayeri AA, et al. Comparison of magnetic resonance angiography and (18)F-fluorodeoxyglucose positron emission tomography in large-vessel vasculitis. Ann Rheum Dis 2018;77:1165–71.

31. Tso E, Flamm SD, White RD, et al. Takayasu arteritis: utility and limitations of magnetic resonance imaging in diagnosis and treatment. Arthritis Rheum 2002;46: 1634–42.

32. Saadoun D, Vautier M, Cacoub P. Medium- and Large-Vessel Vasculitis. Circulation 2021;143:267–82.

33. Chung SA, Gorelik M, Langford CA, et al. 2021 American College of Rheumatology/Vasculitis Foundation Guideline for the Management of Polyarteritis Nodosa. Arthritis Care Res (Hoboken) 2021;73:1061–70.

34. Chung SA, Gorelik M, Langford CA, et al. 2021 American College of Rheumatology/Vasculitis Foundation Guideline for the Management of Polyarteritis Nodosa. Arthritis Rheumatol 2021;73:1384–93.

35. Mukhtyar C, Guillevin L, Cid MC, et al. EULAR recommendations for the management of primary small and medium vessel vasculitis. Ann Rheum Dis 2009;68: 310–7.

36. Guillevin L, Cohen P, Mahr A, et al. Treatment of polyarteritis nodosa and microscopic polyangiitis with poor prognosis factors: a prospective trial comparing glucocorticoids and six or twelve cyclophosphamide pulses in sixty-five patients. Arthritis Rheum 2003;49:93–100.

37. Ombrello AK, Qin J, Hoffmann PM, et al. Treatment Strategies for Deficiency of Adenosine Deaminase 2. N Engl J Med 2019;380:1582–4.

38. Chung SA, Langford CA, Maz M, et al. 2021 American College of Rheumatology/ Vasculitis Foundation Guideline for the Management of Antineutrophil Cytoplasmic Antibody-Associated Vasculitis. Arthritis Rheumatol 2021;73:1366–83.

39. Chung SA, Langford CA, Maz M, et al. 2021 American College of Rheumatology/ Vasculitis Foundation Guideline for the Management of Antineutrophil Cytoplasmic Antibody-Associated Vasculitis. Arthritis Care Res (Hoboken) 2021;73: 1088–105.

40. Yates M, Watts RA, Bajema IM, et al. EULAR/ERA-EDTA recommendations for the management of ANCA-associated vasculitis. Ann Rheum Dis 2016;75:1583–94.

41. Walsh M, Merkel PA, Peh CA, et al. Plasma Exchange and Glucocorticoids in Severe ANCA-Associated Vasculitis. N Engl J Med 2020;382:622–31.

42. Furuta S, Nakagomi D, Kobayashi Y, et al. Effect of Reduced-Dose vs High-Dose Glucocorticoids Added to Rituximab on Remission Induction in ANCA-Associated Vasculitis: A Randomized Clinical Trial. JAMA 2021;325:2178–87.

43. Jayne DRW, Merkel PA, Schall TJ, et al. Avacopan for the Treatment of ANCA-Associated Vasculitis. N Engl J Med 2021;384:599–609.

44. de Groot K, Harper L, Jayne DR, et al. Pulse versus daily oral cyclophosphamide for induction of remission in antineutrophil cytoplasmic antibody-associated vasculitis: a randomized trial. Ann Intern Med 2009;150:670–80.

45. Stone JH, Merkel PA, Spiera R, et al. Rituximab versus cyclophosphamide for ANCA-associated vasculitis. N Engl J Med 2010;363:221–32.

46. Jones RB, Tervaert JW, Hauser T, et al. Rituximab versus cyclophosphamide in ANCA-associated renal vasculitis. N Engl J Med 2010;363:211–20.

47. Jayne DR, Gaskin G, Rasmussen N, et al. Randomized trial of plasma exchange or high-dosage methylprednisolone as adjunctive therapy for severe renal vasculitis. J Am Soc Nephrol 2007;18:2180–8.

48. Springer JM, Kalot MA, Husainat NM, et al. Granulomatosis With Polyangiitis and Microscopic Polyangiitis: A Systematic Review and Meta-Analysis of Benefits and Harms of Common Treatments. ACR Open Rheumatol 2021;3:196–205.

49. Guillevin L, Pagnoux C, Karras A, et al. Rituximab versus azathioprine for maintenance in ANCA-associated vasculitis. N Engl J Med 2014;371:1771–80.

50. Pagnoux C, Mahr A, Hamidou MA, et al. Azathioprine or methotrexate maintenance for ANCA-associated vasculitis. N Engl J Med 2008;359:2790–803.

51. Gopaluni S, Smith RM, Lewin M, et al. Rituximab versus azathioprine as therapy for maintenance of remission for anti-neutrophil cytoplasm antibody-associated vasculitis (RITAZAREM): study protocol for a randomized controlled trial. Trials 2017;18:112.

52. Charles P, Terrier B, Perrodeau E, et al. Comparison of individually tailored versus fixed-schedule rituximab regimen to maintain ANCA-associated vasculitis remission: results of a multicentre, randomised controlled, phase III trial (MAINRIT-SAN2). Ann Rheum Dis 2018;77:1143–9.

53. Kitching AR, Anders HJ, Basu N, et al. ANCA-associated vasculitis. Nat Rev Dis Primers 2020;6:71.
54. Menditto VG, Rossetti G, Olivari D, et al. Rituximab for eosinophilic granulomatosis with polyangiitis: a systematic review of observational studies. Rheumatology (Oxford) 2021;60:1640–50.
55. Wechsler ME, Akuthota P, Jayne D, et al. Mepolizumab or Placebo for Eosinophilic Granulomatosis with Polyangiitis. N Engl J Med 2017;376:1921–32.

Treatment Guidelines in Pediatric Rheumatic Diseases

Ekemini A. Ogbu, MD, MSc[a,b,*], Hermine I. Brunner, MD, MBA[a]

KEYWORDS

- Guideline • Treatment • Rheumatology • Pediatrics

KEY POINTS

- Treatment guidelines in pediatric rheumatology are limited to only a few diseases.
- Stronger evidence studies are needed to inform guidelines for pediatric rheumatic diseases.
- There is a need for regular revision of treatment guidelines.
- Creation of treatment guidelines for rarer pediatric rheumatic diseases would likely improve patient outcomes through consistent consideration of available medical evidence in patient diagnosis, surveillance, and treatment.

INTRODUCTION

Pediatric rheumatologists manage a spectrum of chronic autoimmune, autoinflammatory, and noninflammatory musculoskeletal disorders. Most of these disorders are uncommon or rare.[1,2] Treatment guidelines provide references for clinical practice, while also aiding in directing health policy, and providing a framework for health resource allocation. They are intended to be recommendations and do not substitute clinician judgment.[3]

Treatment guidelines are derived from the best available scientific evidence. Broadly, the intent is to provide guidance to clinicians, and inform best practices. Optimally, evidence stems from well-conducted randomized clinical trials (RCTs), systematic reviews, and meta-analyses. However, the rarity of pediatric rheumatology diseases limits the feasibility of conducting controlled studies. Generally, only a single RCT is performed in support of the efficacy and safety of a new medication, and active comparator studies are exceedingly uncommon. As such, treatment guidelines in

---
[a] Cincinnati Children's Medical Center and University of Cincinnati, Johns Hopkins University, 3333 Burnet Avenue, MLC 4010, Cincinnati, OH 45229, USA; [b] Department of Pediatrics, Johns Hopkins University, Baltimore, Maryland, USA
* Corresponding author.
E-mail address: ekemini.ogbu@cchmc.org

Rheum Dis Clin N Am 48 (2022) 725–746
https://doi.org/10.1016/j.rdc.2022.03.007
0889-857X/22/© 2022 Elsevier Inc. All rights reserved.

pediatric rheumatology often consider lower-grade available evidence, which could include expert opinion, case reports or other observational studies, and use extrapolation of evidence from adult studies.

Published treatment guidelines in pediatric rheumatology are limited to a few diseases. The principal ones are for juvenile idiopathic arthritis (JIA), systemic lupus erythematosus (SLE), uveitis, juvenile dermatomyositis (JDM), systemic vasculitides, and autoinflammatory disorders. Although there may be regional and national differences in recommendations, there are overlapping themes and suggestions.

Methodology of Clinical Guideline Development for Pediatric Rheumatic Diseases

The American College of Rheumatology (ACR) has supported the development of clinical practice guidelines for some pediatric rheumatic diseases. These guidelines have been derived through a meticulous process that involves determining the disease or topic priority, and openly inviting interested parties and stakeholders. This includes pediatric rheumatologists in different practice settings, patient advocates, and relevant organizations. The convened guideline development team completes a systematic review, and the grading of recommendations assessment, development, and evaluation (GRADE) methodology is used in determining the level of evidence to inform the strength of recommendations.[4–6]

In contrast, the Childhood Arthritis and Rheumatology Research Alliance (CARRA) has developed consensus treatment plans (CTPs) for 9 pediatric rheumatic diseases in North America.[7] CTPs differ from treatment guidelines in that the aim is to allow for the conduct of Comparative Effectiveness Studies. The CARRA CTPs are standardized treatment regimens derived through consensus methodology. CTP development is an investigator-initiated process that begins by identifying the clinical problem, determining the existing variability in treatment, and then outlining treatment strategies with perceived comparable treatment benefits. Unlike treatment guidelines that are based on the best available evidence for the disease, CTPs are based on treatment practices in the community, which may not always correspond to the best level of available scientific evidence.

The Single Hub and Access point for pediatric Rheumatology in Europe (SHARE) initiative was started in 2012 with the aim of providing care and treatment recommendations for children with rheumatic diseases in Europe. Participating centers belong to the Pediatric Rheumatology International Trials Organization and the Pediatric Rheumatology European Society (PRES). The SHARE guidelines use the European League Against Rheumatism (EULAR)-standardized operating procedures for the elaboration, evaluation, dissemination, and implementation of recommendation methodology.[8] Recommendations are derived via systematic reviews, Delphi surveys, and consensus methodology. Similar to the GRADE methodology, available evidence is categorized and the strength of recommendation determined by the category of evidence **(Table 1)**.

Given the rapidly advancing science and therapeutic options, regular updates to treatment guidelines seem warranted. It is crucial to keep treatment guidelines updated in order to maintain their value in clinical practice and avoid endorsement of outdated medical evidence. The frequency of guideline revisions vary and updates every 3 to 5 years has been suggested.[9,10] Within the ACR, the Practice Guidelines Subcommittee and the Quality of Care Committee review existing guidelines annually for the need for revision. An example may be the 2011 treatment guideline for JIA, which was revised in 2013. CARRA aims to review its CTPs every 3 years to determine if changes should be made. Although this revision timeline has not been consistently followed, changes may include modification to a treatment arm, addition of a new

Table 1

Comparison of the Grading of Recommendations Assessment, Development and Evaluation and European League against Rheumatism standardized operating procedures for the elaboration, evaluation, dissemination, and implementation of recommendation methodology

Methodology	Categories of Evidence	Strength of Recommendation
GRADE	High quality (A): implies that further research is unlikely to change confidence in the initially estimated effect of an intervention	1—Strong[a] recommendation FOR using an intervention
	Moderate quality (B): implies that further research may have an important impact and may likely change confidence in the initially estimated effect of an intervention	1—Strong recommendation AGAINST using an intervention
	Low quality (C): implies that further research will very likely have an important impact and will likely change confidence in the initially estimated effect of an intervention	2—Weak or conditional[b] recommendation FOR using an intervention
	Very-low quality (D): implies that any estimate of effect of the intervention is very uncertain	2—Weak or conditional recommendation AGAINST using an intervention
EULAR-standardized operating procedures	1A: Obtained from meta-analysis of randomized controlled trials	A—Based on category I evidence
	1B: Obtained from at least one RCT	B—Based on category II evidence or extrapolated from category I evidence
	2A: Obtained from at least one controlled study without randomization	C—Based on category III evidence or extrapolated from category I or II evidence
	2B: Obtained from at least one type of quasi-experimental study	D—Based on category IV evidence or extrapolated from category II or III evidence
	3: Obtained from descriptive studies	
	4: Obtained from expert opinions or committee reports	

[a] Strong recommendations imply that the benefits of an intervention clearly outweigh or do not outweigh the risks.
[b] Weak recommendations imply that it is unclear whether the benefits of an intervention outweigh the risks.

Original tables using previously published data: Data from Guyatt GH, Oxman AD, Kunz R, et al. Going from evidence to recommendations. Bmj. May 10 2008;336(7652):1049-51; Guyatt GH, Oxman AD, Vist GE, et al. GRADE: an emerging consensus on rating quality of evidence and strength of recommendations. Bmj. Apr 26 2008;336(7650):924-6 and Dougados M, Betteridge N, Burmester GR, et al. EULAR standardised operating procedures for the elaboration, evaluation, dissemination, and implementation of recommendations endorsed by the EULAR standing committees. Ann Rheum Dis. Sep 2004;63(9):1172-6.

treatment arm, deletion of a treatment arm, or retraction of an entire CTP.[11] No updates to the SHARE guidelines have occurred. Additionally, there is a continued need for real-world appraisal of derived treatment guidelines.[12,13]

The goal of this review is to give an overview of current and past treatment guidelines in pediatric rheumatology, discuss approaches to deriving these guidelines, demonstrate the need for consistent revision of guidelines, and the need to develop guidelines for other rare diseases in pediatric rheumatology.

Therefore, we conducted a PubMed search of treatment guidelines for the more common pediatric rheumatology conditions from 1966 till December 2021. We also performed a manual Internet search for professional rheumatology society guidelines in the United States and other countries.

DISCUSSION
Juvenile Idiopathic Arthritis

JIA is the most common rheumatologic condition in children. It occurs worldwide with an incidence of 1.6 to 23/100,000, and prevalence of 1 to 4/1000 children.[14] JIA is defined as chronic arthritis of at least 6 weeks duration and with the onset of arthritis before the age of 16 years. It is composed of a heterogeneous group of chronic arthritides. The current classification of JIA is based on the International League of Associations for Rheumatology (ILAR) classification derived in 1995 and modified in 2004.[15] There are 7 subtypes, which include rheumatoid factor positive, rheumatoid factor negative, oligo articular, juvenile psoriatic arthritis, enthesitis-related arthritis, systemic JIA (sJIA), and undifferentiated arthritis.

The first ACR treatment guidelines for JIA were published in 2011.[10] Using the Research and Development/University of California at Los Angeles (RAND/UCLA) Appropriateness method, and the Appraisal of Guidelines for Research and Evaluation instrument, guidance on the initiation and safety monitoring of antirheumatic medications including corticosteroids, nonsteroidal anti-inflammatory drugs (NSAIDS), biologic and nonbiologic disease modifying drugs (DMARDS) was provided. Rather than using the ILAR JIA classification, 5 treatment groups were derived. They are (1) history of arthritis of 4 or fewer joints, (2) history of arthritis of 5 or more joints, (3) active sacroiliitis, (4) systemic arthritis with active systemic features and no active arthritis, and (5) systemic arthritis with active arthritis. The 2011 JIA guidelines provided recommendations on the use of intra-articular corticosteroid injection, duration of NSAID monotherapy, and timing of initiation of Tumor Necrosis Factor inhibitor (TNFi) treatment. Methotrexate was deemed inappropriate for the initial management of a patient with sJIA and fever but without active arthritis. In 2013, these ACR guidelines were updated, given the results of clinical trials and heightened insights in the pathoetiology of JIA.[16]

The 2013 guideline iteration specifically addressed the use of biologic and nonbiologic DMARD treatment in sJIA. This included the use of antiinterleukin 1 (IL-1) and anti-IL-6 therapies and differential recommendations for sJIA treatment based on the presence or absence of active systemic features and arthritis, respectively. Additionally, guidance was given for sJIA patients whose disease is complicated by Macrophage Activation syndrome (MAS). Anakinra was recommended as an initial therapy for sJIA patients with systemic features but not rilonacept, although both medications act on the IL-1 pathway. Notably, corticosteroid or NSAID monotherapy were both limited to a maximum of 1 month for sJIA, and both were deemed inappropriate for initial sJIA therapy. Recommended subsequent therapy for continued sJIA disease activity included canakinumab, tocilizumab, and in the setting of ongoing active sJIA despite the aforementioned biologic DMARDs, the use of the CTLA4 inhibiting biologic DMARD, abatacept. Calcineurin inhibitors were suggested for patients with continued systemic features without active synovitis, after a trial of IL-1 inhibitor and/or tocilizumab. Initiation of methotrexate or leflunomide was recommended for sJIA patients with active joint counts despite the use of IL-1 inhibition or tocilizumab. TNFi were also recommended in this scenario. Treatment with rituximab was deemed mostly inappropriate in both initial and continued disease scenarios with sJIA.[17] In 2015, these treatment recommendations were adopted by the Canadian Rheumatology Association for management of JIA with some modifications for their patient population.[18]

In 2018, a EULAR convened task force provided recommendations for the concept of targeted therapy in JIA.[19] By consensus methodology, it was agreed that the treatment strategy and therapy decisions should be shared between the pediatric rheumatology team and the patient/family. This tailored treat-to-target approach involves setting the treatment target, deciding on JIA monitoring tools, and therapeutics based on individual patient characteristics and patient/family input. It was determined that goals of JIA treatment included controlling disease features, preventing structural damage and comorbidities, and optimizing function and quality of life. Achievement of inactive disease or a low disease activity state with JIA is the most common treatment targets.

In 2019, the ACR revised their recommendations for the treatment of JIA (nonsystemic polyarticular JIA, sacroiliitis, and enthesitis).[14] This covered recommendations for the use of NSAIDs, conventional DMARDs, biologic DMARDs, oral and intra-articular corticosteroids as initial therapy, continued therapy, adjunct therapy, and general use (**Table 2**). The GRADE methodology was newly used rather than the RAND/UCLA methodology for prior JIA guidelines developed by the ACR. Unfortunately, the supporting evidence for 90% of the recommendations were low to very low in quality. Recommendations given included for the use of NSAIDs as adjunct therapy only, the preferred use of subcutaneous methotrexate over oral methotrexate, and methotrexate over leflunomide or sulfasalazine, the use of intra-articular corticosteroid injection as adjunct therapy, and preferred initial therapy with a conventional DMARD over a biologic DMARD. Conventional DMARDs were strongly recommended over NSAID monotherapy, the use of triamcinolone hexacetonide over triamcinolone acetonide for intra-articular injection, and a combination of infliximab with a conventional DMARD. Physical and occupational therapy were recommended for all those children at risk of or with functional limitations.

The first consensus recommendation for the treatment of any pediatric rheumatic disease in less resourced countries (LRC) was for JIA in 2018. There was strong agreement that the management of JIA should be multidisciplinary and best done by clinicians skilled in caring for this disease. They addressed unique challenges of LRC in managing JIA. This included consideration for differential diagnoses (such as malignancies, sickle cell disease, and endemic infections such as tuberculosis, chikungunya, and human immune deficiency syndrome) and specific recommendations on timing of live immunizations in patients on immune suppression.[20]

Juvenile Idiopathic Arthritis-Associated Uveitis

Uveitis is the most frequent extra-articular complication of JIA and can result in irreversible vision loss. In 10% to 20% of patients with JIA, this presents as chronic anterior uveitis (CAU) but the progression to panuveitis may occur.[21–23] CAU is associated with few or no symptoms, and antinuclear antibody (ANA)-positive patients with oligoarticular JIA subtype are at the highest risk of developing CAU. Conversely, acute

Table 2
Current treatment guidelines for juvenile idiopathic arthritis and juvenile idiopathic arthritis-associated uveitis from the American College of Rheumatology

Disease (Year of Publication)	Statements (Level of Evidence)	Strength of recommendation	Previous Versions
JIA[a]	In patients with nonsystemic polyarthritis:		2011 and 2013
(Nonsystemic polyarthritis, sacroiliitis, and enthesitis) (2019)	Use of triamcinolone hexacetonide is strongly recommended over triamcinolone acetonide (B)	1	
	Use of combination therapy with a DMARD is strongly recommended for infliximab (C)	1	
	Use of initial therapy with a DMARD is strongly recommended over NSAID monotherapy (B)	1	
	NSAIDs are conditionally recommended as adjunct therapy (D)	2	
	Use of MTX is conditionally recommended over leflunomide or sulfasalazine (B for MTX, D for sulfasalazine)	2	
	Use of subcutaneous MTX is conditionally recommended over oral MTX (D)	2	
	Use of intra-articular corticosteroids is conditionally recommended as adjunct therapy (D)	2	
	Use of bridging course of oral corticosteroids (<3 mo) is conditionally recommended during initiation or escalation of therapy in patients with high or moderate disease activity (D)	2	
	Initially starting biologics, combination therapy with a DMARD is conditionally recommended over biologic monotherapy (D for etanercept and	2	

(continued on next page)

Table 2 (continued)			
Disease (Year of Publication)	Statements (Level of Evidence)	Strength of recommendation	Previous Versions
	golilumab, C for abatacept and tocilizumab, B for adalimumab)		
	Use of MTX monotherapy as initial therapy is conditionally recommended over triple DMARD therapy (C)	2	
	PT and/or OT is conditionally recommended for JIA patients who are at risk of/or have functional limitations (C for PT, D for OT)	2	
	Initial therapy with a DMARD is conditionally recommended over a biologic in patients without risk factors (C)	2	
	Use of DMARD as initial therapy is conditionally recommended over a biologic in patients with risk factors (C)	2	
	Escalation of therapy is conditionally recommended over no escalation of therapy in patients with polyarthritis refractory to a DMARD or biologic (D)	2	
	With refractory arthritis (moderate or high disease activity) despite DMARD monotherapy, adding a biologic is conditionally recommended over switching to a second DMARD (C)	2	
	With moderate or high disease activity on DMARD monotherapy, adding a biologic is conditionally recommended over switching to triple DMARD therapy (C)	2	

(continued on next page)

Table 2
(continued)

Disease (Year of Publication)	Statements (Level of Evidence)	Strength of recommendation	Previous Versions
	With refractory arthritis (moderate or high disease activity) on a first TNFi (with or without a DMARD), switching to a non-TNFi biologic is conditionally recommended over switching to a second TNFi (D)	2	
	With refractory arthritis (moderate or high disease activity) on a second biologic, switching to TNFi, abatacept or tocilizumab is conditionally recommended over rituximab (D)	2	
	Use of chronic corticosteroids regardless of disease activity and risk factors is strongly recommended against (D)	1	
	Conditionally recommend against use of bridging course of oral corticosteroids (<3 mo) in patients with low disease activity (D)	2	
	In patients with JIA and sacroiliitis:		
	Use of an NSAID is strongly recommended over no treatment with an NSAID, in the presence of active sacroiliitis (D)	1	
	Addition of a TNFi is strongly recommended over NSAID monotherapy, in the presence of continued active sacroiliitis while on NSAIDs		
	With active sacroiliitis despite NSAID use, and who have failed more than one TNFi or have contraindications to	2	

(continued on next page)

Table 2
(continued)

Disease (Year of Publication)	Statements (Level of Evidence)	Strength of recommendation	Previous Versions
	TNFi, using sulfasalazine is conditionally recommended (C)		
	With active sacroiliitis despite NSAID use, bridging therapy with short oral corticosteroid course (<3 mo) during initiation or escalation of therapy is conditionally recommended (D)	2	
	With active sacroiliitis despite NSAID use, intra-articular corticosteroid injection of the sacroiliac joints is conditionally recommended as adjunct therapy (D)	2	
	PT is conditionally recommended for those who are at risk of functional limitations (D)	2	
	With active sacroiliitis despite NSAID use, methotrexate monotherapy is strongly recommended against (D)	1	
	In patients with JIA and enthesitis:		
	With active enthesitis, use of NSAIDs is strongly recommended over no treatment with an NSAID (D)	1	
	With active enthesitis despite NSAID use, starting a TNFi is conditionally recommended over methotrexate or sulfasalazine (C)	2	
	With active enthesitis despite NSAID use, a bridging short course of oral corticosteroids (<3 mo is conditionally recommended (D)	2	

(continued on next page)

Table 2 (continued)			
Disease (Year of Publication)	**Statements (Level of Evidence)**	**Strength of recommendation**	**Previous Versions**
	PT is conditionally recommended for those who have, or at risk of functional limitations (D)	2	
JIA associated uveitis (2019)[a]	Ophthalmic screening every 3 mo is conditionally recommended for patients with JIA at high risk of developing uveitis (C)	2	None
	For patients with JIA and controlled uveitis undergoing tapering or discontinuation of topical glucocorticoids, eye examinations within 1 mo of each change is strongly recommended (D)	1	
	In patients with JIA and controlled uveitis on stable therapy, eye examinations at least every 3 mo is strongly recommended (D)	1	
	In patients with JIA and controlled uveitis undergoing tapering or discontinuation of systemic therapy glucocorticoids, eye examinations within 2 mo of changing systemic therapy is strongly recommended (D)	1	
	In patients with JIA and active CAU, use of prednisolone acetate 1% topical drops in conditionally recommended over difluprednate topical drops (D)	2	
	In patients with JIA and active CAU, short-term addition or increase in topical corticosteroid drops is conditionally	2	

(continued on next page)

Table 2 (continued)			
Disease (Year of Publication)	Statements (Level of Evidence)	Strength of recommendation	Previous Versions
	recommended over adding systemic corticosteroids (D)		
	In patients with JIA with new-onset CAU activity despite being on stable systemic therapy, trial of topical corticosteroids is conditionally recommended over changing/escalating systemic therapy immediately (D)	2	
	In patients with JIA and CAU still needing 1–2 drops/d of prednisolone acetate 1% (or equivalent) for uveitis control, and not on systemic therapy, addition of systemic therapy is conditionally recommended over maintaining on topical corticosteroids only (D)	2	
	In patients with JIA and CAU on systemic therapy, and still needing 1–2 drops/d of prednisolone acetate 1% (or equivalent) for at least 3 mo, changing or escalating systemic therapy is conditionally recommended over maintaining same systemic therapy (D)	2	
	In patients with JIA and CAU initiating systemic therapy for uveitis, use of subcutaneous methotrexate is conditionally recommended over oral methotrexate (D)	2	
	In patients with JIA and severe active CAU and sight-threatening complications, initiating methotrexate plus a	2	

(continued on next page)

Table 2
(continued)

Disease (Year of Publication)	Statements (Level of Evidence)	Strength of recommendation	Previous Versions
	monoclonal TNFi (adalimumab or infliximab) immediately is conditionally recommended over methotrexate monotherapy (D)		
	In patients with JIA and active CAU starting a TNFi, a monoclonal TNFi is conditionally recommended over etanercept (D)	2	
	In patients with JIA and active CAU refractory to 1 monoclonal TNFi at standard dose, escalating the dose and/or frequency is conditionally recommended over switching to other TNFi (D)	2	
	In patients with JIA and active CAU refractory to 1 monoclonal TNFi above standard dose/frequency, switching to other monoclonal TNFi is conditionally recommended over other category of biologic therapy (D)	2	
	In patients with JIA and active CAU refractory to methotrexate and 2 monoclonal antibody TNFi, at above-standard dose and/or frequency, other biologic therapy options (abatacept or tocilizumab) or nonbiologic therapy (mycophenolate, leflunomide, or cyclosporine) are conditionally recommended (D)	2	
	Education on warning signs of AAU is strongly	1	

(continued on next page)

Table 2
(continued)

Disease (Year of Publication)	Statements (Level of Evidence)	Strength of recommendation	Previous Versions
	recommended for JIA patients with spondyloarthritis (D)		
	In patients with JIA and spondyloarthritis controlled on systemic immunosuppression (biologic and/or nonbiologic DMARDS), who develop AAU, trial of topical steroids is conditionally recommended over switching to other systemic immunosuppression immediately (D)	2	
	In patients with JIA and CAU controlled on systemic therapy but still on 1–2 drops/d of prednisolone acetate 1% (or equivalent), tapering topical glucocorticoids first is strongly recommended over tapering systemic steroid first (D)	1	
	In patients with JIA and uveitis who are well controlled on biologic therapy and DMARD, at least 2 y of well-controlled disease is conditionally recommended before tapering (D)	2	

Abbreviations: AAU, acute anterior uveitis; CAU, chronic anterior uveitis; DMARD, disease modifying antirheumatic drug; NSAID, nonsteroidal anti-inflammatory drugs; OT, occupational therapy; PT, physical therapy; TNFi, tumor necrosis factor inhibitor.

[a] Guidelines were derived using the GRADE methodology. Level of evidence: B—moderate quality, C—low quality, D—very low quality. Strength of recommendation: 1—strong recommendation, that is, desirable effects of an intervention clearly outweigh the undesirable effect, 2—conditional recommendation, that is, when it is unclear if the intervention outweighs the undesirable effects.

Original Tables using previously published data: Data from Ringold S, Angeles-Han ST, Beukelman T, et al. 2019 American College of Rheumatology/Arthritis Foundation Guideline for the Treatment of Juvenile Idiopathic Arthritis: Therapeutic Approaches for Non-Systemic Polyarthritis, Sacroiliitis, and Enthesitis. Arthritis Care and Research. 2019/6// 2019;71(6):717-734 and Angeles-Han ST, Ringold S, Beukelman T, et al. 2019 American College of Rheumatology/Arthritis Foundation Guideline for the Screening, Monitoring, and Treatment of Juvenile Idiopathic Arthritis–Associated Uveitis. Arthritis Care and Research. 2019/6// 2019;71(6):703-716.

anterior uveitis (AAU) is associated with HLA B27 positivity, enthesitis-related arthritis, and JPsA.

The 2018 SHARE recommendations provided the first international guidance on JIA-associated uveitis. These recommendations were derived using the EULAR-standardized operating procedures.[8] The aim of the guidelines was to offer recommendations to prevent or decrease the risk of uveitis, inform strategies in support of earlier uveitis diagnosis to prevent damaging sequelae, and guide treatment strategies. SHARE uveitis recommendations include having continuous communication between treating ophthalmologist and pediatric rheumatologist regarding management, and immediate initiation of treatment of active uveitis. Topical ocular corticosteroids were recommended as first-line treatment. Systemic immune suppression was recommended if there is still active uveitis 3 months postinitiation of ocular corticosteroids or if there was reactivation of uveitis during the tapering of corticosteroids. Methotrexate was recommended as the initial systemic therapy for active CAU, and TNFi (adalimumab, infliximab, and golimumab) for methotrexate-resistant disease. Second-line uveitis treatments recommended for TNFi refractory disease included tocilizumab, rituximab, and abatacept. Notably, etanercept was deemed to be ineffective for uveitis treatment and should not be used.[23]

In 2019, the ACR derived recommendations for JIA-associated uveitis using the GRADE methodology.[22] Similar to the SHARE guidelines, communication between the managing rheumatologist and ophthalmologist was strongly recommended. Patients and family should be educated about warning signs of AAU. It was also recommended that patients with JIA and controlled uveitis should have at least 3 monthly eye examinations, and at least within 1 month of tapering or discontinuing corticosteroids. Conditional recommendations included that in severe CAU and/or sight-threatening complications, start of combination therapy of methotrexate plus a TNFi was preferred to methotrexate monotherapy. Overall, the recommendations were mostly based on low-quality level of evidence, highlighting the need for controlled studies with adequate number of study subjects (see **Table 2**).

Systemic Lupus Erythematosus

SLE is the second most common rheumatic disease in childhood. The annual incidence of childhood-onset SLE (cSLE) is 0.3 to 0.9/100,000, and the prevalence is 1.89 to 25.7/100,000.[24] cSLE is a vastly phenotypically heterogeneous disease, associated with significant morbidity and mortality.

Using the EULAR-standardized operating procedures, the SHARE initiative guidelines for cSLE diagnosis and treatment was published in 2017.[24,25] Recommendations included that the most severe clinical feature of cSLE should guide treatment decisions. Use of the Systemic Lupus International Collaborating Clinics SLE classification criteria was recommended to enable early recognition, and referral to pediatric specialists for cSLE evaluation, and initiation of therapy was endorsed. Further, the ACR nomenclature and case definition for neuropsychiatric features should be used in classifying neuropsychiatric lupus in pediatric patients.

Recommendations regarding diagnostics included obtaining a chest X-ray and screening for cardiac abnormalities at diagnosis of cSLE. Investigation for respiratory features without an infectious source should include a pulmonary function test (PFT) with diffusing capacity of lung for carbon monoxide (DLCO). Infection and MAS should be considered in patients with cSLE and fever. Annual eye examinations while on hydroxychloroquine were recommended.

In general, patients with cSLE should have regular disease activity monitoring using a standardized disease activity measure, and standardized damage assessment annually. Monitoring of patients with active cSLE should include a full clinical evaluation every 2 to 4 weeks for 2 to 4 months after a flare, or following a new cSLE diagnosis.

Children with cSLE requiring chronic corticosteroid use should be monitored for linear growth. Brain imaging was recommended but it was recognized that the imaging may be normal despite neuropsychiatric lupus. Cognitive function with cSLE should be monitored using validated tests such as the Pediatric Automated Neuropsychological Assessment Metrics or formal neuropsychological testing. Treatment of all patients with cSLE should include hydroxychloroquine, and conventional DMARDs added to the treatment regimen when corticosteroids cannot be tapered. Some examples of conventional DMARDs for cSLE treatment included mycophenolate mofetil (MMF), azathioprine, cyclophosphamide, and methotrexate.

The Latin American Group for the Study of Lupus (GLADEL) and the Pan-American League of Associations for Rheumatology (PANLAR) developed treatment recommendation and guidelines for SLE in 2018.[26] Some of the recommendations were specific for cSLE and aligned with the SHARE recommendations.

In 2012, EULAR and the European Renal Association European Dialysis and Transplant Association the issued joint recommendations for the management of lupus nephritis in children and adults.[27] The EULAR-standard operating procedures and the Appraisal of Guidelines Research and Evaluation Instrument were used in deriving the guideline statements. For both children and adults, MMF or cyclophosphamide in combination with corticosteroids was recommended for proliferative lupus nephritis. MMF with corticosteroids was recommended for pure membranous lupus nephritis with nephrotic range proteinuria. Rituximab or a calcineurin inhibitor was recommended for refractory membranous nephritis. This is similar to the 2017 SHARE recommendations for lupus nephritis in children but differs from the GLADEL/PANLAR recommendation for high-dose corticosteroids plus MMF or cyclophosphamide for induction therapy for lupus nephritis in general.[26,28] CARRA-derived CTPs for the treatment of proliferative lupus nephritis during the initial 6 months; there are 3 corticosteroid dosing strategies and 2 alternatives for steroid-sparing immune suppression, that is, MMF or cyclophosphamide.[29]

Juvenile Dermatomyositis

JDM is a rare disease with an annual incidence of 2 to 4/million children.[30,31] However, it is the most common idiopathic inflammatory myopathy in children and associated with dermatopathic and vasculopathic changes. In some cases, there is pulmonary involvement and development of calcinosis but cardiac involvement is even rarer.

The SHARE initiative developed the treatment guidelines for JDM in 2016. Seven overarching principles and 59 recommendations were derived with 66% of the recommendations based on expert opinion[30]: Recommendations included that children with JDM should be managed at centers with expertise with caring for this disease. Magnetic resonance imaging (MRI) could be used for diagnosis but an open muscle biopsy was indicated when JDM presentation is atypical. Muscle ultrasound was an option when muscle biopsy could not be done or MRI was unavailable. Measurement of myositis specific antibodies and myositis-associated antibodies were recommended. An assessment of swallow function and evaluation for pulmonary involvement, ECHO, and EKG should all be done at diagnosis. Disease monitoring should include the use of standardized measures such as the Childhood Myositis Assessment Scale.

Treatment goals should include disease control, prevention of damage, improved quality of life, and physical activity. Treatment induction regimen should include high-dose corticosteroids (intravenous or oral) and methotrexate. For patients with methotrexate intolerance, MMF or cyclosporine may be used. With inadequate JDM response to the initial 12 weeks of induction therapy or emergence of calcinosis, escalation of therapy should be considered. For refractory disease, MMF, rituximab, and TNFi medications may be used. Infliximab and adalimumab are preferred over etanercept. Intravenous immunoglobulin can be considered as adjunctive therapy for refractory disease. For treatment of severe JDM with major end-organ involvement or ulcerative skin disease, intravenous cyclophosphamide is a recommended treatment option.

Serum biomarkers, such as muscle enzymes measurements, and MRI can be used for monitoring of myositis. Disease surveillance should include monitoring for the development of calcinosis. Recommended adjunct therapies for JDM include photoprotection, occupational therapy, and physical therapy. Given the absence of a single diagnostic test that can establish the diagnosis of JDM with 100% specificity, alternative diagnoses should be considered for patients who lack cutaneous signs and/or fail to respond to therapy as expected. Based on expert consensus only, it was recommended that withdrawal of therapy may be considered in patients who successfully discontinued corticosteroids and remained in remission on methotrexate or another DMARD for at least 1 year.

Juvenile scleroderma

Juvenile scleroderma encompasses 2 broad categories, juvenile systemic scleroderma (JSSc) and juvenile localized scleroderma (JLS). The latter is often limited to the skin and subdermal tissues, whereas extracutaneous involvement is rare. JLS subcategories include circumscribed morphea, linear scleroderma, generalized morphea, pansclerotic morphea, and a mixed JLS subtype.

In 2019, consensus-based recommendations for JLS were published by the SHARE initiative. These recommendations focused on the assessment of skin disease, and extracutaneous involvement, and treatment pathways at disease onset and with refractory course. The JLS guidelines recommend that all children with suspected JLS should be referred to a specialized pediatric rheumatology center for evaluation and management. Further, JLS course should be monitored using validated outcome measures. The Localized Scleroderma Skin Damage Index and the Localized Scleroderma Skin Severity Index were considered the best-suited clinical tools for the assessment of skin damage and disease activity/severity, respectively. Infrared thermography and specialized ultrasound imaging with Doppler use were thought to be useful in assessing disease activity. MRI should be considered for musculoskeletal assessment, particularly when a JLS skin lesion crosses a joint. In patients with face and head involvement, brain MRI should be done at the time of diagnosis, irrespective of the presence or absence of neurologic involvement. Routine surveillance of a child with JLS should comprise a complete joint examination that includes the temporomandibular joint; as well as orthodontic and maxillofacial evaluations. Further, uveitis screening should be done at diagnosis, and regular follow-up eye examinations are recommended, particularly for children with face, head, and neck disease. All JLS experts concurred that oral or intravenous pulse-dose corticosteroid regimens may be used to treat active disease, and that methotrexate or other conventional DMARDs should be started at the same time as systemic corticosteroids. Subcutaneous or oral methotrexate at dosages of 15 mg/m^2/wk was recommended and tapering should only occur with clinical improvement and after a minimum of 12 months of methotrexate use. MMF can be used alone, or in combination with methotrexate, for refractory JLS treatment. Experts recommended ultraviolet A1 phototherapy and topical imiquimod to improve skin thickening in circumscribed lesions.[32]

The SHARE initiative also resulted in consensus-based recommendations for JSSc that were published in 2021.[33] It was recommended that all children with suspected

JSSc be treated at a specialized pediatric rheumatology center. Patients with isolated Raynaud phenomenon and abnormal nailfold capillaroscopy and/or ANA positivity should have regular follow-up. JSSc monitoring using a standardized skin score tool was recommended such as the JSSc Severity Score (J4S) or the modified Rodnan skin score, despite the fact that this index has not undergone formal validation for use in pediatrics. SHARE experts recommended that JSSc surveillance should occur every 6 months and include PFT with DLCO, cardiac echocardiogram, renal function, and completion of the modified Rodnan skin score. PFT with DLCO are sensitive tools for detecting and monitoring interstitial lung disease. Regarding treatment, conventional DMARDs, especially methotrexate, should be started at the time of JSSc diagnosis and used for the treatment of active JSSc. Treatment of active JSSc also involves systemic corticosteroid, and MMF or other conventional DMARD may be used for refractory disease. Pulmonary and cardiac involvement should be treated with cyclophosphamide, and for severe or refractory disease, biologic DMARDs such as rituximab and tocilizumab may be used. In some instances of refractory disease, autologous stem cell transplantation (HSCT) may be considered. The synthetic analog of prostacyclin PGI2, iloprost, can be used for the treatment of digital ischemia and ulcerations, and bosetan, a dual endothelin receptor antagonist, can be added for refractory disease or severe pulmonary hypertension.

Both the JLS and JSSc consensus guidelines' strength of recommendations is limited by the lack of high-level or strong medical evidence, for example, limited data on the validity of pediatric tools for skin and overall severity assessment, benefits of HSCT, and data supporting the efficacy of MMF, biologic DMARDs and antifibrotic agents in JSSc, for example, nintedanib.

Systemic Vasculitides

Systemic vasculitides are a heterogeneous group of autoimmune disorders in which blood vessel inflammation is the predominant feature. These rare disorders are often classified using the 2006 EULAR/PRES classification criteria for childhood vasculitis and, or the 2012 revised International Chapel Hill Consensus on Nomenclature of Systemic Vasculitides.[34,35]

Pediatric-specific treatment guidelines for systemic vasculitides are scarce. To address this, in 2018, the SHARE initiative derived consensus-based recommendations for treatment and diagnosis.[36] This included recommendations for childhood polyarteritis nodosa (PAN), granulomatosis with polyangiitis, eosinophilic granulomatosis with polyangiitis, and Takayasu arteritis derived from available small descriptive pediatric studies, or adult studies providing moderate-to-high level scientific evidence. Recommendations include a stepwise diagnostic approach, considering differential diagnoses such as infections, monogenic autoinflammatory diseases, and malignancies, and importantly, determining the extent of organ involvement. It was noted that enzyme-linked immunosorbent assay, plus immunofluorescence, is the preferred approach to measuring antineutrophil cytoplasmic antibodies. Disease monitoring should include the pediatric vasculitis activity score. Although tissue biopsy is desirable, the lack thereof should not preclude the initiation of emergent or life-threatening disease. Depending on disease severity, induction therapy for vasculitis includes high-dose or pulse corticosteroids, intravenous cyclophosphamide, plasmapheresis, and/or biologic DMARDs. Standard maintenance treatment includes azathioprine, methotrexate, MMF, or biologic DMARDs particularly rituximab. For PAN, TNFi and IL-6 blockade are additional recommended maintenance options. It was advised that therapy withdrawal only be considered after the completion of a minimum of 12 months of maintenance therapy.

Autoinflammatory Disorders

Autoinflammatory disorders comprise a range of diseases in which there is primarily dysregulation of the innate immune system. These disorders may be monogenic or polygenic and have overlapping autoimmune features or immune deficiency. The best-defined autoinflammatory rheumatic diseases are cryopyrin-associated periodic fever syndrome (CAPS), mevalonate kinase deficiency (MVKD), and TNF receptor-associated periodic syndrome (TRAPS). CAPS is a spectrum of disorders caused by gain-of-function mutations in the *NLRP3* gene. These include familial cold autoinflammatory syndrome, Muckle-Wells syndrome, and neonatal-onset multisystem inflammatory disease (also known as chronic infantile neurologic, cutaneous, and articular syndrome). Chronic recurrent multifocal osteomyelitis (CRMO), also known as chronic nonbacterial osteomyelitis is a rare autoinflammatory bone disease. Although sJIA may be considered an autoinflammatory disease, recommendations for sJIA are included in that of other categories of JIA.

Given the scarcity of evidence, treatment guidelines exist for only a few of these autoinflammatory disorders. There are the 2015 SHARE recommendations for the treatment and monitoring of autoinflammatory disorders focusing on CAPS, MVKD, and TRAPS.[37] These were derived using the EULAR standard operating procedure methodology.[8] Recommendations include a multidisciplinary approach to the management of patients with autoinflammatory disorders with care best provided at a tertiary center with experts in treating these diseases and available genetic counseling. Shared decision-making of the medical team, and the patient and family-centered care is considered ideal and should include psychosocial support.

For treatment of CAPS, IL-1 inhibition is indicated at any age and early initiation of the treatment in patients with active disease is recommended. There is no evidence of efficacy of conventional DMARDs or other biologic DMARDs besides IL-1 inhibitors in CAPS. For treatment of TRAPS, IL-1 inhibition is effective in most cases, and although etanercept and corticosteroids are effective, therapeutic benefits may wane over time. For treatment of MVKD, short-term IL-1 inhibition is recommended during episodes of active inflammation. Long-term IL-1 blockade or etanercept are recommended for frequent inflammatory attacks or persistent subclinical inflammation. Colchicine and statins are not recommended for MVKD and allogeneic HSCT may be considered in severe refractory disease and poor quality of life. NSAIDs and corticosteroids can be used as adjuvant symptomatic therapy but not as primary maintenance therapy for CAPS, MVKD, and TRAPS. The reliance on low-level strength of evidence is a strong limitation of this guideline.

There are no treatment guidelines for CRMO but CARRA developed a CTP for the initial 12 months after diagnosis.[38] Three treatment arms with comparable effectiveness for CRMO disease refractory to NSAIDs and/or with active spine involvement were established: (1) monotherapy with methotrexate or sulfasalazine, (2) use of a TNFi (adalimumab, etanercept, and infliximab) with or without methotrexate, and (3) bisphosphonates, specifically pamidronate or zoledronic acid. A significant limitation of this CTP is that recommendations for therapy arms were based mostly on common clinical practice habits, expert opinion, and evidence from mostly small observational studies.

SUMMARY

In summary, we gave an overview of treatment guidelines in pediatric rheumatology. We emphasized the benefits of treatment guidelines in enhancing evidence-based care in general. We discussed the limitations of the current guidelines in pediatric rheumatology and the need for stronger evidence studies to inform guidelines. The limitations in the strength of evidence for each pediatric rheumatic disease condition are almost universal.

Because of the limited available scientific evidence, there is a reliance on extrapolation of adult data and guidelines for the management of pediatric rheumatic diseases. Although this may be advantageous as an interim measure, it is recognized that this is not ideal. This is because pediatric-onset diseases such as SLE tend to be more severe, and the disease biology may not always directly correlate with adult-onset disease. Hence optimal treatment regimens could differ from adult-onset disease. Furthermore, adult guidelines are often inadequate in addressing other aspects of caring for a child with chronic illness such as psychosocial considerations and mitigating the impact of the disease and medications on growth, development, and outcomes in adulthood. Additionally, rheumatic diseases which are predominantly of pediatric onset are not often addressed by adult guidelines. An example of this is the monogenic autoinflammatory syndromes.

Overall, there is a need for continued development and consistent revision of treatment guidelines for pediatric rheumatic diseases. There is need to expand the scope to include other rare rheumatic diseases.

CLINICS CARE POINTS

- Although the use of treatment guidelines is voluntary, the guidelines provide evidence-based approaches for managing diseases to improve outcomes.
- Several treatment guidelines (eg, for juvenile idiopathic arthritis, systemic lupus erythematosus, juvenile dermatomyositis, and autoinflammatory disorders) emphasize that where available, children with rheumatic diseases are best cared for at specialized centers with a pediatric rheumatologist.
- Where available, the use of standardized monitoring tools is recommended for pediatric rheumatic diseases.

DISCLOSURE

E.A. Ogbu has nothing to disclose. H.I. Brunner has nothing to disclose that is relevant to this article.

REFERENCES

1. Schaller JG. The history of pediatric rheumatology. Pediatr Res 2005;58(5): 997–1007.
2. Woo P, Colbert RA. An overview of genetics of paediatric rheumatic diseases. Best Pract Res Clin Rheumatol 2009;23(5):589–97.
3. Pai M, Iorio A, Meerpohl J, et al. Developing methodology for the creation of clinical practice guidelines for rare diseases: A report from RARE-Bestpractices. Rare Dis 2015;3(1):e1058463.
4. Barbar-Smiley F, Ashley Cooper MPH, Edelheit B, et al. American College of Rheumatology (ACR) Juvenile Idiopathic Arthritis Guideline Literature Review Team. Available at: https://www.rheumatology.org/Portals/0/Files/JIA-Guideline-Project-Plan-2021.pdf.
5. Guyatt GH, Oxman AD, Kunz R, et al. Going from evidence to recommendations. BMJ 2008;336(7652):1049–51. AE.

6. Guyatt GH, Oxman AD, Vist GE, et al. GRADE: an emerging consensus on rating quality of evidence and strength of recommendations. BMJ 2008;336(7650): 924–6. AD.

7. Ringold S, Nigrovic PA, Feldman BM, et al. The childhood arthritis and rheumatology research alliance consensus treatment plans: toward comparative effectiveness in the pediatric rheumatic diseases. Arthritis Rheumatol 2018;70(5): 669–78.

8. Dougados M, Betteridge N, Burmester GR, et al. EULAR standardised operating procedures for the elaboration, evaluation, dissemination, and implementation of recommendations endorsed by the EULAR standing committees. Ann Rheum Dis 2004;63(9):1172–6.

9. Vernooij RW, Sanabria AJ, Solà I, et al. Guidance for updating clinical practice guidelines: a systematic review of methodological handbooks. Implement Sci 2014;9:3.

10. Beukelman T, Patkar NM, Saag KG, et al. American College of Rheumatology recommendations for the treatment of juvenile idiopathic arthritis: initiation and safety monitoring of therapeutic agents for the treatment of arthritis and systemic features. Arthritis Care Res (Hoboken) 2011;63(4):465–82.

11. Policy for Revising an Approved CARRA Consensus Treatment Plan. Available at: https://carragroup.org/UserFiles/file/CTPRevisionProcedures_Approved2021.06.28.pdf.

12. Smith CAM, Toupin-April K, Jutai JW, et al. A systematic critical appraisal of clinical practice guidelines in juvenile idiopathic arthritis using the appraisal of guidelines for research and evaluation II (AGREE II) instrument. PLoS One 2015;10(9).

13. Kimura Y, Grevich S, Beukelman T, et al. Pilot study comparing the childhood arthritis & rheumatology research alliance (carra) systemic juvenile idiopathic arthritis consensus treatment plans. Pediatr Rheumatol 2017;15(1).

14. Ringold S, Angeles-Han ST, Beukelman T, et al. American college of rheumatology/arthritis foundation guideline for the treatment of juvenile idiopathic arthritis: therapeutic approaches for non-systemic polyarthritis, sacroiliitis, and enthesitis. Arthritis Care Res 2019;71(6):717–34.

15. Petty RE, Southwood TR, Manners P, et al. International League of Associations for Rheumatology classification of juvenile idiopathic arthritis: second revision, Edmonton, 2001. J Rheumatol 2004;31(2):390–2.

16. Ringold S, Weiss PF, Beukelman T, et al. 2013 update of the 2011 American college of rheumatology recommendations for the treatment of juvenile idiopathic arthritis: Recommendations for the medical therapy of children with systemic juvenile idiopathic arthritis and tuberculosis screening among children receiving biologic medications. Arthritis Care Res 2013;65(10):1551–63.

17. Ringold S, Weiss PF, Beukelman T, et al. 2013 update of the 2011 American College of Rheumatology Recommendations for the treatment of juvenile idiopathic arthritis: Recommendations for the medical therapy of children with systemic juvenile idiopathic arthritis and tuberculosis screening among children receiving biologic medications. Arthritis Rheum 2013;65(10):2499–512.

18. Cellucci T, Guzman J, Petty RE, et al. Management of juvenile idiopathic arthritis 2015: a position statement from the pediatric committee of the canadian rheumatology association. J Rheumatol 2016 Oct;43(10):1773–6.

19. Ravelli A, Consolaro A, Horneff G, et al. Treating juvenile idiopathic arthritis to target: recommendations of an international task force. Ann Rheum Dis 2018; 77(6):819–28.

20. Scott C, Chan M, Slamang W, et al. Juvenile arthritis management in less re-sourced countries (JAMLess): consensus recommendations from the Cradle of Humankind. Clin Rheumatol 2019;38(2):563–75.
21. Angeles-Han ST, Lo MS, Henderson LA, et al. Childhood arthritis and rheuma-tology research alliance consensus treatment plans for juvenile idiopathic arthritis–Associated and idiopathic chronic anterior uveitis. Arthritis Care Res 2019;71(4):482–91.
22. Angeles-Han ST, Ringold S, Beukelman T, et al. American College of rheuma-tology/arthritis foundation guideline for the screening, monitoring, and treatment of juvenile idiopathic arthritis–associated uveitis. Arthritis Care Res 2019;71(6): 703–16.
23. Constantin T, Foeldvari I, Anton J, et al. Consensus-based recommendations for the management of uveitis associated with juvenile idiopathic arthritis: The SHARE initiative. Ann Rheum Dis 2018;77(8):1107–17.
24. Groot N, De Graeff N, Avcin T, et al. European evidence-based recommendations for diagnosis and treatment of childhood-onset systemic lupus erythematosus: The SHARE initiative. Ann Rheum Dis 2017;76(11):1788–96.
25. Smith EMD, Sen ES, Pain CE. Diagnosis and treatment of childhood-onset sys-temic lupus erythematosus (European evidence-based recommendations from the SHARE initiative). In: Abbasi K, editor. Archives of disease in childhood: ed-ucation and practice edition. London: BMJ Publishing Group; 2019. p. 259–64.
26. Pons-Estel BA, Bonfa E, Soriano ER, et al. First Latin American clinical practice guidelines for the treatment of systemic lupus erythematosus: Latin American Group for the Study of Lupus (GLADEL, Grupo Latino Americano de Estudio del Lupus)-Pan-American League of Associations of Rheumatology (PANLAR). Ann Rheum Dis 2018;77(11):1549–57.
27. Bertsias GK, Tektonidou M, Amoura Z, et al. Joint european league against rheu-matism and european renal association-european dialysis and transplant associ-ation (EULAR/ERA-EDTA) recommendations for the management of adult and paediatric lupus nephritis. Ann Rheum Dis 2012;71(11):1771–82.
28. Groot N, De Graeff N, Marks SD, et al. European evidence-based recommenda-tions for the diagnosis and treatment of childhood-onset lupus nephritis: The SHARE initiative. Ann Rheum Dis 2017;76(12):1965–73.
29. Mina R, Von Scheven E, Ardoin SP, et al. Consensus treatment plans for induction therapy of newly diagnosed proliferative lupus nephritis in juvenile systemic lupus erythematosus. Arthritis Care Res 2012;64(3):375–83.
30. Enders FB, Bader-Meunier B, Baildam E, et al. Consensus-based recommenda-tions for the management of juvenile dermatomyositis. Ann Rheum Dis 2017; 76(2):329–40.
31. Huber AM, Giannini EH, Bowyer SL, et al. Protocols for the initial treatment of moderately severe juvenile dermatomyositis: results of a Children's arthritis and rheumatology research alliance consensus conference. Arthritis Care Res (Hobo-ken) 2010;62(2):219–25.
32. Zulian F, Culpo R, Sperotto F, et al. Consensus-based recommendations for the management of juvenile localised scleroderma. Ann Rheum Dis 2019;78(8): 1019–24.
33. Foeldvari I, Culpo R, Sperotto F, et al. Consensus-based recommendations for the management of juvenile systemic sclerosis. Rheumatology (Oxford) 2021; 60(4):1651–8.
34. Schnabel A, Hedrich CM. Childhood vasculitis. Frontiers in pediatrics. Switzerland: Frontiers Media S.A.; 2019.

35. Ozen S, Ruperto N, Dillon MJ, et al. EULAR/PReS endorsed consensus criteria for the classification of childhood vasculitides. Ann Rheum Dis 2006;65(7):936–41.
36. De Graeff N, Groot N, Brogan P, et al. European consensus-based recommendations for the diagnosis and treatment of rare paediatric vasculitides-the SHARE initiative. Rheumatology (United Kingdom) 2019;58(4):656–71.
37. Ter Haar NM, Oswald M, Jeyaratnam J, et al. Recommendations for the management of autoinflammatory diseases. Ann Rheum Dis 2015;74(9):1636–44.
38. Zhao Y, Wu EY, Oliver MS, et al. Consensus treatment plans for chronic nonbacterial osteomyelitis refractory to nonsteroidal antiinflammatory drugs and/or with active spinal lesions. Arthritis Care Res 2018;70(8):1228–37.

The Evaluation of Guideline Quality in Rheumatic Diseases

Claire E.H. Barber, MD, PhD, FRCPC[a,b,c,*],
Cheryl Barnabe, MD, MSc, FRCPC[a,b,c],
Nicole M.S. Hartfeld, MSc, MC, CCC[b], Kiran Dhiman, MPH[b],
Glen S. Hazlewood, MD, PhD, FRCPC[a,b,c]

KEYWORDS

- Rheumatology • Practice guideline • Evidenced-based medicine • Implementation
- Quality of care

KEY POINTS

- Strategies for meaningful patient engagement in guideline development are evolving and should be implemented to improve the incorporation of evidence from studies of patient preferences into guidelines.
- Health equity considerations were lacking in most reviewed guidelines, even those that used the Grading of Recommendations Assessment, Development, and Evaluation methodology.
- Transparent strategies for implementing and documenting editorial independence of rheumatology guideline panels could be improved for most guidelines.
- Implementation strategies for guidelines were infrequently described but sometimes effectively deployed by rheumatology societies; however, link to guidelines could be described more clearly.

INTRODUCTION

Guidelines for the management of rheumatic diseases have been developed by rheumatology organizations and societies globally to direct clinicians to apply high quality and evidence-driven care for patients with rheumatic diseases in their practices, assist in developing quality monitoring programs, and advocate for access to treatment and

[a] Department of Medicine, Cumming School of Medicine, University of Calgary, 2500 University Dr NW, Calgary, AB T2N 1N4, Canada; [b] Department of Community Health Sciences, Cumming School of Medicine, University of Calgary, 2500 University Dr NW, Calgary, AB T2N 1N4, Canada; [c] Arthritis Research Canada, 2238 Yukon St, #230, Vancouver, BC V5Y 3P2, Canada
* Corresponding author. 3280 Hospital Drive Northwest, HMRB Building, Room 451, Calgary, Alberta T2N 4N1, Canada.
E-mail address: cehbarbe@ucalgary.ca

Rheum Dis Clin N Am 48 (2022) 747–761
https://doi.org/10.1016/j.rdc.2022.03.008
rheumatic.theclinics.com

other health resources. The methods used in guideline development vary by organization and have evolved over time. While some organizations develop new guidelines on a regular basis, others adopt or adapt guidance[1] from other larger organizations for both efficiency and contextualization for local implementation.[2–4] The Grading of Recommendations Assessment, Development, and Evaluation (GRADE) approach[5] is becoming increasingly accepted as the standard for transparent guideline development internationally.

Guideline quality is commonly appraised using the international Appraisal of Guidelines for Research and Evaluation (AGREE) II instrument.[6] The instrument includes six domains assessing the rigor and transparency of guideline development including: scope and purpose; stakeholder involvement; rigor of development; clarity of presentation; applicability; and editorial independence (**Table 1**). Each domain includes multiple items, which are rated on a Likert scale from 1 (strongly disagree) to 7 (strongly agree) using a standardized checklist. Beyond item scores and domain scores, an overall quality score for the guideline is ascertained from 1 (lowest possible quality) to 7 (highest possible quality) as well as an overall recommendation for use (yes, yes with modifications, no). Recently, the Appraisal of Guidelines for Research and Evaluation – Recommendations Excellence (AGREE-REX) has been developed as a complement to the AGREE II.[7] Where the primary focus of the AGREE II is the quality of the guideline development process, the AGREE-REX evaluates the quality of the guideline recommendations.[7] Health equity, which has been more recently emphasized in GRADE methodology,[8] is not explicitly addressed in the AGREE II. The AGREE-REX, however, includes items to assess the guidelines consideration of patient values and preferences and the description of how to tailor recommendations for diverse patient populations.

Our aim is to appraise and discuss the quality of selected major rheumatology guidelines using the AGREE II instrument. The scope of our review was English-language guidelines published in the last 5 years from major international rheumatology societies with a focus on the treatment of inflammatory arthritis, vasculitides, and systemic lupus erythematosus and related conditions. Given the breadth of

Table 1
Appraisal of Guidelines for Research and Evaluation II domains

Domain	Types of Items Included*
Scope and Purpose	The objective(s), health question(s), and target population(s) of the guideline are specifically described
Stakeholder Involvement	The relevant professional groups, target population (eg, patients), and target users of the guideline are involved in its development
Rigor of Development	The evaluation of evidence and development and grading recommendations is systematic, transparent, clearly linked and has undergone external review by experts
Clarity of Presentation	Key recommendations are clear, specific, and easy to identify
Applicability	The guideline offers a discussion of facilitators and barriers to its implementation (including resource implications), alongside advice and tools to facilitate implementation and evaluation criteria
Editorial Independence	Conflicts of interest (including the funding body) are disclosed and addressed

*For complete list of items within each domain see reference[6]

rheumatological conditions included, we focused on assessing the overall guideline development process with the AGREE II and did not evaluate the quality of individual guideline recommendations with the AGREE-REX. However, as the AGREE II tool has limitations, we also included an evaluation of the use of GRADE methodology and reviewed how health equity was addressed in rheumatology guideline development.

Guideline Quality

The AGREE II ratings for each of the 16 evaluated guidelines are shown in **Table 1**. We included guidelines for gout, lupus, psoriatic arthritis and spondylarthritis, rheumatoid arthritis (RA), and vasculitis from five major societies. Overall, seven guidelines from the American College of Rheumatology (ACR) and Australian Rheumatology Association (ARA) used the GRADE method, and an additional two reported some variation/ modification of the GRADE method. The following sections present the findings of our review by the elements suggested in the AGREE II and an additional evaluation of how health equity considerations were incorporated into major rheumatology guidelines.

Stakeholder involvement

The AGREE II instrument includes three items in this domain capturing whether the guideline development group includes individuals from all the relevant professional groups, whether patients' views and preferences have been sought, and that the target guideline users are clearly defined. In this domain, the area of major variability was patient involvement in the guideline development process. Although 15 of the 16 reviewed guidelines explicitly mentioned inclusion of patients on the guideline panels, there was variability in the number of individuals including how input was sought and how it was presented and incorporated into guidelines. An example of how differences in the inclusion of patients may impact recommendations was identified in the recent gout guidelines from the ACR[9] and European Alliance of Associations for Rheumatology (EULAR).[10] Since a 2016 study investigating the feasibility of developing recommendations based on a patient panel,[11] ACR guideline development has involved a separate patient panel reviewing the evidence and providing patient perspectives for consideration by the guideline voting panel.[12] The ACR 2020 gout guidelines[9] were developed using a GRADE approach and included an in-person panel of eight male patients with gout. They reviewed the evidence in a moderated discussion with a voting panel member and provided patient preferences and perspectives. The core voting panel also included a patient representative. Both initial guideline questions and final recommendations were also posted for public comment. Several of the ACR gout guideline recommendations provided clear discussion of how patient input had impacted the voting panel. In contrast, while there was patient representation ($n = 2$) on the voting panel for the EULAR guidelines, it was unclear how patient input was considered when making recommendations besides patients casting a vote for their level of agreement with the final recommendations.[10]

Beyond the inclusion of patient representatives on guideline panels, the GRADE approach recommends a systematic and transparent approach for incorporating patient values and preferences in the guideline development. Evidence may be incorporated systematically in the Evidence to Decision (EtD) framework (**Box 1**) from several types of sources including both qualitative and quantitative studies.[13] Current guidance from the Australian Living Guideline on the management of inflammatory arthritis do transparently discuss patient preferences in their EtD framework (although data are limited to a single qualitative study).[14] No other guidelines systematically sought evidence on patient preferences in their EtD process.

> **Box 1**
> **Overview of the grading of recommendations assessment, development, and evaluation evidence to decision framework**
>
> - The EtD framework provides a systematic and transparent process for moving from evidence to guideline panel decisions. The structure of the framework consists of three main elements: question formulation, assessment of evidence, and drawing conclusions.
> - Question formulation requires a structured format describing the Problem, Intervention, Comparison, and Outcomes (PICO).
> - Assessment of the evidence is facilitated by summary findings tables which are concise summaries of research evidence for each important outcome, the magnitude of the effect of the intervention, and a judgment regarding the certainty of the evidence.
> - To facilitate transparency when drawing conclusions from the evidence, the EtD also summarizes the evidence and panel judgments related to several domains that are considered when deciding on the direction and strength of the recommendation, including any uncertainty/variability in how much individuals value the main outcomes, balance of effects (between desirable and undesirable effects), resources required and certainty of evidence of resources required, cost effectiveness, impact on health equity, acceptability to key stakeholders, and feasibility of implementation.
> - A summary of judgments table is often used to concisely display the evidence from all domains in a matrix.
> - Panels review the assessment of the evidence, consider the implications, develop actionable recommendations, and draw conclusions about the direction and strength of each recommendation.
>
> *Data from* Alonso-Coello P, Schünemann HJ, Moberg J, Brignardello-Petersen R, Akl EA, Davoli M, Treweek S, Mustafa RA, Rada G, Rosenbaum S, Morelli A, Guyatt GH, Oxman AD; GRADE Working Group. GRADE Evidence to Decision (EtD) frameworks: a systematic and transparent approach to making well informed healthcare choices. 1: Introduction. BMJ. 2016 Jun 28;353:i2016.

Rigor of development

The AGREE II instrument includes eight items within this domain. Ratings of reviewed guidelines are shown in **Table 2**. Although the AGREE II instrument does not explicitly align with the GRADE methodology, we noted higher AGREE II ratings in this domain for guidelines that used the GRADE approach to develop recommendations. We suggest this may have been due to the guideline developers' adherence to the clear and transparent process recommended by GRADE through the use of the EtD framework. For example, the ACR and ARA guidelines used the GRADE approach and included tables presenting the findings from the evaluation of evidence quality; thus, those guidelines scored highly for presenting a process that clearly linked the supporting evidence to each recommendation. In contrast, guidelines that did not use the GRADE approach often did not clearly describe how the quality of evidence was evaluated nor present findings from such an evaluation. Therefore, these guidelines received lower AGREE II ratings in this domain due to the insufficient transparency of the process.

A noteworthy difference in the process of finalizing recommendations was observed when comparing ACR and EULAR guidelines. ACR recommendations require at least 70% consensus among panel members to be included in the final guidelines. In contrast, in the standardized operating procedures (SOPs) for EULAR-endorsed recommendations,[15] there is no requisite minimal level of consensus. Of the EULAR guidelines reviewed, percent agreement between voting panel members was above

Table 2
Appraisal of guidelines for research and evaluation II domain scores and overall guideline assessment

Organization (Year, Guideline)	Scope and Purpose	Stakeholder Involvement	Rigor of Development	Clarity of Presentation	Applicability	Editorial Independence	Overall Quality Rating—Recommended for Use[a]
Inflammatory Arthritis							
Australian Living Guideline for Inflammatory Arthritis (2021)	100%	100%	97%	100%	87%	100%	7—Recommended without modification
ACR (2021, RA)	100%	88%	87.5%	100%	54%	100%	6—Recommended with modifications
EULAR (2019, RA)	61%	44%	47%	100%	20%	66%	4—Recommended with modifications
ACR (2020, Gout)	94%	83%	91%	94%	41%	100%	6—Recommended with modifications
EULAR (2016, Gout)	94%	77%	62%	61%	12%	66%	4—Recommended with modifications
EULAR (2019, PsA)	83%	61%	39%	100%	20%	66%	4—Recommended with modifications
ACR (2018, PsA)	100%	83%	91%	100%	41%	100%	6—Recommended with modifications
GRAPPA (2015, PsA)	100%	83%	39%	61%	45%	33%	4—Recommended with modifications
Vasculitides							
ACR (2021, PAN)	100%	88%	91%	100%	41%	100%	6—Recommended with modifications
ACR (2021, GCA and TAK)	100%	83%	91%	100%	33%	100%	6—Recommended with modifications
ACR (2021, ANCA-Associated Vasculitis)	100%	88%	91%	100%	37%	100%	6—Recommended with modifications

(continued on next page)

Table 2
(continued)

Organization (Year, Guideline)	Scope and Purpose	Stakeholder Involvement	Rigor of Development	Clarity of Presentation	Applicability	Editorial Independence	Overall Quality Rating—Recommended for Use[a]
CanVasc (2020, ANCA-Associated Vasculitis)	100%	72%	93%	88%	20%	66%	5—Recommended with modifications
EULAR (2016, ANCA-Associated Vasculitis)	100%	77%	87%	94%	45%	58%	6—Recommended with modifications
EULAR (2018, LVV)	100%	83%	77%	88%	20%	75%	5—Recommended with modifications
SLE and Related Conditions							
EULAR (2019, SLE)	88%	16%	68%	77%	12%	66%	4—Recommended with modifications
EULAR (2019, LN)	100%	83%	60%	72%	12%	66%	5—Recommended with modifications

Guidelines are grouped disease type, and within that, guidelines from different organizations regarding the same disease are grouped together and organized by year (newest to oldest). AGREE II items were scored from 1 (Strongly Disagree) to 7 (Strongly Agree). Domain percentages were calculated by adding the scores of all items in a domain, dividing the sum by the highest possible score for the domain and multiplying by 100.

Abbreviations: ACR, American College of Rheumatology; AGREE II, Appraisal of Guidelines for Research and Evaluation II; ANCA, antineutrophil cytoplasmic antibody; CanVasc, Canadian Vasculitis Research Network; EULAR, European Alliance for Associations for Rheumatology; GCA, giant cell arteritis; GRAPPA, Group for Research and Assessment of Psoriasis and Psoriatic Arthritis; LN, lupus nephritis; LVV, large vessel vasculitis; PAN, polyarteritis nodosa; PsA, psoriatic arthritis; RA, rheumatoid arthritis; SLE, systemic lupus erythematosus; TAK, Takayasu arteritis.

[a] Overall quality rating is the assessor's judgment of the overall quality of the guideline from 1 (Lowest Possible Quality) to 7 (Highest Possible Quality). Recommended for Use is the assessor's judgment on whether or not the guidelines are recommended for use, with the following options: Yes (use the guideline as is), Yes with modifications or No (do not recommend guideline for use).

80% for six out of seven guidelines. However, in the EULAR, recommendations for management of antineutrophil cytoplasmic antibody (ANCA)-associated vasculitis consensus were as low as 53% with eight statements less than 70% agreement.[16] As EULAR SOPs instruct recommendation strength is based on the Oxford Levels of Evidence—which categorizes evidence based on the type of research design, with the highest category being meta-analysis of randomized controlled trials (RCTs)—even recommendations with less than 70% agreement can be strongly recommended.[15] In the EULAR ANCA-associated vasculitis guideline, three statements are given the highest strength of recommendation (A), despite less than 60% agreement among panel members.[16]

Two additional items in the AGREE II domain of rigor of development consistently received lower ratings in our evaluation that the guideline is externally reviewed by experts and a procedure for updating the guideline is provided. External review by experts refers to a process of formal consultations with experts (including methodologists) and potentially the patient/public external to the guideline development panel. There is little specification in the AGREE II instrument as to the optimal number of external reviewers, how to receive feedback and how to adequately and transparently incorporate feedback received. The ACR has outlined a process for feedback through review and approval of guidelines by multiple sources including journal peer review, ACR Guideline Subcommittee, ACR Quality of Care Committee, and ACR Board of Directors Review, and public comment.[12] What was less clear among all guidelines were explicitly how feedback was collected (eg, simply comments or response to specific questions vs approval) and where feedback was recorded and incorporated in guidelines when elicited (such documents appeared often internal). Where and how public comment is solicited may also be challenging and may not always offer opportunity for meaningful public engagement. Furthermore, the number, type of reviewers, and affiliations were often unclear, leading to lower ratings for many guidelines on this item.

The frequency of updating guidelines also varied. The current ACR strategy for determining when to update a guideline is to update literature searches periodically (ideally quarterly) and for the results to be screened by ACR guidelines subcommittee and staff, potentially with expert input. A series of "signals"[17] are used to evaluate whether there are major changes in the evidence base, which could change recommendations based on research evaluating how quickly systematic reviews become out of date.[17] Examples of new evidence which may change guidance include: new high quality large RCTs; new meta-analyses (with at least one new trial not previously considered); new RCTs when prior guidance only based on observational data; important changes in effectiveness; expansion of treatment; and important caveats (eg, about patient populations who may benefit, increases in harm, etc.).[12] Given the potential for different interpretations of what qualifies as a "signal" warranting a guideline update, there was a slight downgrading of ratings on this item for ACR guidelines. Like the approach adopted by ACR, EULAR SOPs do not dictate a specific timeline at which guidelines should be updated. Rather, guideline developers are advised to indicate when it is expected that an update will be necessary. How this is done is open to the best judgment. Unfortunately, many EULAR guidelines omitted mention of the process altogether.

In contrast, an emerging methodology employed by the ARA is that of "Living Guidelines".[14] This strategy leverages systematic reviews with ongoing surveillance for new literature for base recommendations.[18] Elements to this strategy which may differ from standard procedures include continuous surveillance of the literature (in contrast to periodic updates) and incorporation of new data into "living summary tables" as studies are released. This process requires a "living" or "on-call" guideline panel and peer review process.[18] Publication and dissemination of recommendations from this process may differ from standard full-length guideline publications and may include publication of single recommendations that have been modified. Logistically, they may be best disseminated and viewed on online platforms amenable to frequent updates. While we did not explicitly review the quality of COVID-19 vaccination guidelines for rheumatology patients for this review, we have experience with this approach from our Canadian context.[19] Given the rapid development of vaccine efficacy and safety evidence during the pandemic, the living review methodology was found to be extremely useful for developing and updating vaccination guidelines in a seamless fashion. As the conduct of periodic systematic reviews for guideline updates is time-consuming, employment of living reviews methodology may offer an opportunity for collaboration between rheumatology organizations and leveraged by independent societies for local and contextual implementation.

Applicability

Despite the objective of guidelines to inform clinical practice, uptake and implementation remain a challenge.[20–23] There are several strategies that are suggested to improve guideline uptake at policy, institutional, provider, and patient levels.[24] The AGREE II instrument domain on applicability captures these important factors by considering whether the guidelines have described facilitators and barriers to their implementaton, advice, or tools for how the recommendations can be put into practice, resource implications, and monitoring or auditing criteria. Given the practical importance of this domain, it is surprising that most of the guidelines reviewed received low AGREE II ratings. This reflects the frequent lack of discussion about potential barriers/facilitators to implementation and the absence of advice or tools to facilitate implementation.

We identified some organizations that specified clear and effective methods for dissemination and implementation of guidelines. For example, ACR protocols for dissemination include Web site publication (including any interim updates), clinician's guides, pocket guides, or web applications. One important strategy for implementation of guidelines includes the development and implementation of quality measures based on the recommendations. The ACR has developed streamlined strategies for the development of quality measures from guidelines into electronic clinical quality measures.[25] Implementation of the electronic measures in the Rheumatology Informatics System for Effectiveness registry[26,27] supports the ongoing monitoring of care quality and improvements in care in participating practices.

Another strategy to support guideline implementation is the development of patient decision aids and other patient materials to facilitate patient decision-making for preference sensitive treatment choices linked to guidelines.[28] Preference sensitive decisions are ones that require deliberation to carefully weigh risks and benefits according to patient preferences and values.[29] This is a strategy that has not been systematically employed to date in current guidelines of the major organizations that we reviewed with the exception of the ARA.[14]

Editorial independence

While our quality review did not highlight any major concerns about editorial independence of the guideline panels according to the AGREE II criteria, it remains an important consideration and an area of ongoing public interest. While nearly all guidelines had lists of disclosures of interest for panel members, what was sometimes less clear where and how these were managed by the panel during consensus voting. Best practices for managing conflicts of interest have been developed by many societies,[30] and a set of nine principles has been developed by the Guidelines International Network[31]; unfortunately not all of these principles are required in current AGREE II criteria. Current ACR guidance[12] on managing conflict of interests requires the PIs, and literature review leads to be free of conflicts of interest for at least 1 year prior and 1 year following guideline development and publication, and that a minimum of 51% of the panel is conflict of interest free for at least 1 year prior. Similarly, EULAR SOPs[15] require the declaration of potential conflicts of interest before project start; however, the management of conflicts of interest is not further described in this document. An increasingly employed strategy for managing conflicts of interest is for panel members with significant conflicts to recuse themselves from voting on recommendations for which they have potential conflicts.[32] The ARA used a transparent process for managing conflicts of interest. Panel members are assessed as having high, moderate, or low risk of conflicts of interest, and those assessed as high risk do not vote but can contribute to discussion and be authors.[14]

AGREE II overall quality rating
Only the Australian living guidelines[14] received a global rating of "recommend without modification". Due to lower ratings on one or more domains, all other reviewed guidelines were recommended "with modifications" to indicate limitations in development or reporting. **Box 2** describes the strategies we identified to improve guideline quality.

Health equity
Health inequity is defined as differences in health outcomes that are avoidable, unfair, or unjust.[33] The PROGRESS-Plus framework can be used to identify characteristics such as place of residence, occupation, gender/sex, education, and socioeconomic status (among other characteristics), which may result in differential care delivery and outcomes.[34] Although health equity considerations are extremely important to consider when developing and implementing guidelines, they are not explicitly measured in the AGREE II instrument.[35] There is a potential for guidelines to result

---

Box 2
Overview of suggested strategies to address common limitations among guidelines recommended for use with modifications

- Increase involvement of the target population throughout the evidence to decision process and clearly describe how their views and preferences inform guideline development and strength of recommendations.

- Report full search strategies (including search terms, databases, and dates) for the search of the evidence.

- Provide access to a report that summarizes the evaluation of the evidence—including strengths, limitations, risk of bias, and other assessments of certainty—to increase methodological transparency.

- Limit the number of actionable items within each recommendation to one to improve clarity.

- In tables, summarizing key recommendations provide all the information required to understand and appropriately apply recommendations to facilitate application in practice.

- Address guideline implementation and explicitly discuss strategies for applying recommendations in clinical practice.

- Report funding and include a statement addressing conflicts of interest for individuals involved in guideline development.

in intervention-generated inequity, whereby improved outcomes are realized for the general population, but without beneficial impact or even worsening outcomes for those experiencing health inequity.[36] Many of the recent guideline publications from major rheumatology organizations do not appear to explicitly incorporate health equity considerations during development, although some subgroup recommendations are made (**Table 3**). This is an ongoing concern,[35] and guidelines from other organizations including the World Health Organization have also inconsistently incorporated health equity considerations into recommendations.[37]

Table 3
Rating of guidelines for health equity considerations

Organization (Year, Guideline)	Scope and Purpose[a]	Rigor of Development[b]	
Inflammatory Arthritis			
Australian Living Guideline for Inflammatory Arthritis (2021)	7	7	7
ACR (2021, RA)	1	1	3
EULAR (2019, RA)	7	3	7
ACR (2020, Gout)	1	3	2
EULAR (2016, Gout)	1	1	2
EULAR (2019, PsA)	1	1	2
ACR (2018, PsA)	1	3	2
GRAPPA (2015, PsA)	1	3	2
Vasculitides			
ACR (2021, PAN)	1	1	1
ACR (2021, GCA and TAK)	1	2	2
ACR (2021, ANCA-Associated Vasculitis)	1	1	1
CanVasc (2020, ANCA-Associated Vasculitis)	1	3	3
EULAR (2016, ANCA-Associated Vasculitis)	1	3	2
EULAR (2018, LVV)	1	3	2
SLE and Related Conditions			
EULAR (2019, SLE)	1	1	2
EULAR (2019, LN)	1	1	2

Guidelines are grouped disease type, and within that, guidelines from different organizations regarding the same disease are grouped together and organized by year (newest to oldest). Scores presented used a rating system from 1 (strongly disagree) to 7 (strongly agree).

Abbreviations: ACR, American College of Rheumatology; ANCA, antineutrophil cytoplasmic antibody; CanVasc, Canadian Vasculitis Research Network; EULAR, European Alliance for Associations for Rheumatology; GCA, giant cell arteritis; GRAPPA, Group for Research and Assessment of Psoriasis and Psoriatic Arthritis; LN, lupus nephritis; LVV, large vessel vasculitis; PAN, polyarteritis nodosa; PsA, psoriatic arthritis; RA, rheumatoid arthritis; SLE, systemic lupus erythematosus; TAK, Takayasu arteritis.

[a] Scope and purpose regarding health equity is defined as follows: The priorities of disadvantaged groups or populations in relation to the health question(s) covered by the guideline are specifically described.

[b] Rigor of development included two items which were defined as[1] health equity considerations (eg, analysis of differences of effect) in the body of evidence are clearly described[2] and health equity has been considered in formulating the recommendations (eg, balance of likely impact on health equity with other factors). Scores are presented respectively from left to right.

There is a growing interest in this field and an ongoing work in developing strategies for incorporating equity considerations into guidelines and implementation efforts in meaningful ways. The GRADE working group promotes a transparent structured approach, with health equity included as a core criterion in the EtD framework when deciding on strength and direction of recommendations.[38] Additional detailed guidance has been developed.[39–41] However, the logistics of adequately incorporating equity considerations in guideline development and implementation remains an important and emerging field. While the incorporation of equity considerations in guidelines is often included in a separate section of the GRADE EtD framework, many have suggested that it should be considered in all aspects of the framework as it may impact patient preferences, and implementation considerations and how benefits versus harms are perceived and weighed.[42]

Some rheumatology organizations have been working to include equity considerations using the GRADE framework in an explicit and transparent manner.[14] One example includes the Canadian Rheumatology Association (CRA).[42,43] Recently research was conducted to identify potential priority populations who may experience inequities in the implementation of care delivery in the country.[43] While recognizing the intersectionality of individuals' experiences and identities, six priority populations were defined including rural and remote residents, Indigenous Peoples, elderly with frailty, first-generation immigrant and refugee communities, persons with low income and who are vulnerably housed, persons with diversity in sexual orientation and gender identity and expression,[43] and more recently Black Canadians. Through qualitative work with members of these populations of interest and physicians who provide care to them, several contributors to inequity in health service delivery and mitigation approaches were identified for consideration in guideline development and implementation.[43]

From this research, equity considerations relevant to each step in the EtD framework for CRA RA guidelines were then identified.[42] For example, regarding the "priority of the problem" for rural and remote residents, there was a higher priority for questions supporting the logistics of access to care and for elderly persons with frailty on treatment questions focusing on quality of life/symptom control. Major evidence gaps were identified for many of the priority populations related to the magnitude of treatment effect, despite the known potential increased risks of adverse effects and differential opportunity for improvement based on differences in comorbidity profiles; for example, the importance of main outcomes and treatment acceptability may also be different and impacted by other social and cultural factors for some groups. Resource considerations vary between the population groups dependent on drug coverage and employment as examples. Lastly, the feasibility of guideline implementation for different population groups varies based on health system availability and navigation challenges unique to each. For a fulsome discussion of this topic, see Barnabe and colleagues.[42]

A recent example of how this equity framework was incorporated in guideline development includes the CRAs recent guidelines for COVID-19 vaccination in persons with autoimmune rheumatic diseases.[19] Equity considerations are transparently reported in the EtD tables and were considered by the guideline panel and incorporated into the recommendation documentation.[19] The ARA guidelines previously mentioned are another example of clear and transparent inclusion of equity considerations using the GRADE process into recommendations.[14]

Although these efforts to promote health equity in guidelines are encouraging, challenges remain. Many of the trials that guideline recommendations are based on often have underrepresentation of populations experiencing inequities enrolled and do not include assessments of the intervention or treatment in groups representative of all relevant potential populations of interest.[44] For example, trials may exclude populations such as the frail elderly or pregnant women, and there is a limited investigation of treatment effects by socioeconomic groups.[35] While ethical approaches to trial inclusion are defined, observational data may also help inform recommendations in priority populations. Additional qualitative and health system review may be required to get a clear understanding of additional contextual factors which may impact health equity (eg, supply chain, access to care, etc.) for certain populations. Meaningful inclusion of patients on guideline groups or other means of engagement is critical in this process. Lastly, health equity requires a specific focus in implementation efforts,[45] with continuous re-evaluation for disparities emerging and widening, and co-development of solutions to mitigate these with the affected populations.

SUMMARY

GRADE has emerged as the standard for guideline development in rheumatology. More recent elements of the GRADE EtD framework methodology to support health equity and incorporation of patient preferences should become mandatory elements of guideline development. Novel methods such as "living guidelines" offer significant opportunities for collaboration between the guideline groups to maintain timely and seamless guidance. Strategies for implementing guidelines should more clearly discuss at the time of guideline development and may include the parallel development of quality measures and patient decision aids.

CLINICS CARE POINTS

- Consider the rigor of guideline development when selecting guidelines to aid in management of rheumatic disease.
- "Living" guideline recommendations may be available and may be more frequently updated based on best available evidence than traditional guideline publications.
- Review how health equity considerations were incorporated into guidelines and whether these apply to your practice setting and population.
- Consider the use of decision aids and quality measures in your practice to facilitate guideline implementation.

DISCLOSURE

C.E.H. Barber, N.M.S. Hartfeld, K. Dhiman and G. Hazlewood do not have any relevant commercial disclosures. Dr C.E.H. Barber is supported by an Arthritis Society Stars Career Development Award that is funded by the Canadian Institutes of Health Research-Institute of Musculoskeletal Health STAR-19-0611/CIHR SI2-169745. Dr C. Barnabe holds a CIHR Canada Rresearch Chair in Rheumatoid Arthritis and Autoimmune Disease. Dr C. Barnabe has received speaker fees from Pfizer and Sanofi Genzyme and advisory board member fees from Celltrion Healthcare and Gilead. Dr G. Hazlewood is the current Chair of the CRA's Guidelines Committee and Drs C.E.H. Barber and C. Barnabe are members of this committee.

REFERENCES

1. Schunemann HJ, Wiercioch W, Brozek J, et al. GRADE Evidence to Decision (EtD) frameworks for adoption, adaptation, and de novo development of

trustworthy recommendations: GRADE-ADOLOPMENT. J Clin Epidemiol 2017; 81:101–10.

2. Darzi A, Harfouche M, Arayssi T, et al. Adaptation of the 2015 American College of Rheumatology treatment guideline for rheumatoid arthritis for the Eastern Mediterranean Region: an exemplar of the GRADE Adolopment. Health Qual Life Outcomes 2017;15:183.

3. Bykerk VP, Akhavan P, Hazlewood GS, et al. Canadian Rheumatology Association recommendations for pharmacological management of rheumatoid arthritis with traditional and biologic disease-modifying antirheumatic drugs. J Rheumatol 2012;39:1559–82.

4. Mendel A, Ennis D, Go E, et al. CanVasc consensus recommendations for the management of antineutrophil cytoplasm antibody-associated vasculitis: 2020 update. J Rheumatol 2021;48:555–66.

5. Guyatt G, Oxman AD, Akl EA, et al. GRADE guidelines: 1. Introduction-GRADE evidence profiles and summary of findings tables. J Clin Epidemiol 2011;64: 383–94.

6. Brouwers MC, Kho ME, Browman GP, et al. AGREE II: advancing guideline development, reporting and evaluation in health care. CMAJ 2010;182:E839–42.

7. Brouwers MC, Spithoff K, Kerkvliet K, et al. Development and Validation of a Tool to Assess the Quality of Clinical Practice Guideline Recommendations. JAMA Netw Open 2020;3:e205535.

8. Akl EA, Welch V, Pottie K, et al. GRADE equity guidelines 2: considering health equity in GRADE guideline development: equity extension of the guideline development checklist. J Clin Epidemiol 2017;90:68–75.

9. FitzGerald JD, Dalbeth N, Mikuls T, et al. American college of rheumatology guideline for the management of gout. Arthritis Care Res (Hoboken) 2020;72: 744–60.

10. Richette P, Doherty M, Pascual E, et al. 2016 updated EULAR evidence-based recommendations for the management of gout. Ann Rheum Dis 2017;76:29–42.

11. Fraenkel L, Miller AS, Clayton K, et al. When patients write the guidelines: patient panel recommendations for the treatment of rheumatoid arthritis. Arthritis Care Res (Hoboken) 2016;68:26–35.

12. American College of Rheumatology. Policy and procedure manual for clinical practice guidelines. 2015 [updated 2015; cited 2022 January 4th]; Available at: https://www.rheumatology.org/Portals/0/Files/ACR%20Guideline%20Manual_ Appendices_updated%202015.pdf.

13. Zhang Y, Coello PA, Brozek J, et al. Using patient values and preferences to inform the importance of health outcomes in practice guideline development following the GRADE approach. Health Qual Life Outcomes 2017;15:52.

14. ANZMUSC. An Australian living guideline for the pharmacologic management of inflammatory Arthritis [Version 0.3]. 2020. Available at: https://mskguidelines.org.

15. van der Heijde D, Aletaha D, Carmona L, et al. 2014 update of the EULAR standardised operating procedures for EULAR-endorsed recommendations. Ann Rheum Dis 2015;74:8–13.

16. Yates M, Watts RA, Bajema IM, et al. EULAR/ERA-EDTA recommendations for the management of ANCA-associated vasculitis. Ann Rheum Dis 2016;75:1583–94.

17. Shojania KG, Sampson M, Ansari MT, et al. How quickly do systematic reviews go out of date? A survival analysis. Ann Intern Med 2007;147:224–33.

18. Akl EA, Meerpohl JJ, Elliott J, et al. Living systematic review n. living systematic reviews: 4. living guideline recommendations. J Clin Epidemiol 2017;91:47–53.

19. Hazlewood GS, Pardo JP, Barnabe C, et al. Canadian rheumatology association recommendation for the use of covid-19 vaccination for patients with autoimmune rheumatic diseases. J Rheumatol 2021;48:1330–9.

20. Batko B, Batko K, Krzanowski M, et al. Physician adherence to treat-to-target and practice guidelines in rheumatoid arthritis. J Clin Med 2019;8.

21. Lesuis N, van Vollenhoven RF, Akkermans RP, et al. Rheumatologists' guideline adherence in rheumatoid arthritis: a randomised controlled study on electronic decision support, education and feedback. Clin Exp Rheumatol 2018;36:21–8.

22. Lesuis N, den Broeder AA, Hulscher ME, et al. Practice what you preach? An exploratory multilevel study on rheumatoid arthritis guideline adherence by rheumatologists. RMD Open 2016;2:e000195.

23. Ho GH, Pillinger MH, Toprover M. Adherence to gout guidelines: where do we stand? Curr Opin Rheumatol 2021;33:128–34.

24. Chan WV, Pearson TA, Bennett GC, et al. ACC/AHA special report: clinical practice guideline implementation strategies: a summary of systematic reviews by the NHLBI implementation science work group: a report of the american college of cardiology/american heart association task force on clinical practice guidelines. J Am Coll Cardiol 2017;69:1076–92.

25. Yazdany J, Myslinski R, Miller A, et al. Methods for developing the American college of rheumatology's electronic clinical quality measures. Arthritis Care Res (Hoboken) 2016;68:1402–9.

26. Izadi Z, Schmajuk G, Gianfrancesco M, et al. Significant Gains in rheumatoid arthritis quality measures among rise registry practices. Arthritis Care Res (Hoboken) 2022;74:219–28.

27. Yazdany J, Bansback N, Clowse M, et al. The rheumatology informatics system for effectiveness (RISE): a national informatics-enabled registry for quality improvement. Arthritis Care Res (Hoboken) 2016;68:1866–73.

28. Barber CEH, Spencer N, Bansback N, et al. Development of an implementation strategy for patient decision aids in rheumatoid arthritis through application of the behavior change wheel. ACR Open Rheumatol 2021;3:312–23.

29. Elwyn G, Frosch D, Rollnick S. Dual equipoise shared decision making: definitions for decision and behaviour support interventions. Implement Sci 2009;4:75.

30. Traversy G, Barnieh L, Akl EA, et al. Managing conflicts of interest in the development of health guidelines. CMAJ 2021;193:E49–54.

31. Schunemann HJ, Al-Ansary LA, Forland F, et al. Guidelines international network: principles for disclosure of interests and management of conflicts in guidelines. Ann Intern Med 2015;163:548–53.

32. Guyatt G, Akl EA, Hirsh J, et al. The vexing problem of guidelines and conflict of interest: a potential solution. Ann Intern Med 2010;152:738–41.

33. Whitehead M. The concepts and principles of equity and health. Int J Health Serv 1992;22:429–45.

34. O'Neill J, Tabish H, Welch V, et al. Applying an equity lens to interventions: using PROGRESS ensures consideration of socially stratifying factors to illuminate inequities in health. J Clin Epidemiol 2014;67:56–64.

35. Oxman AD, Schunemann HJ, Fretheim A. Improving the use of research evidence in guideline development: 12. Incorporating considerations of equity. Health Res Policy Syst 2006;4:24.

36. White M, Adams J, Heywood P. How and why do interventions that increase health overall widen inequalities within populations?. In: Babones SJ, editor. Social inequality and public health. Bristol: Policy Press; 2009. p. 65–82.

37. Dewidar O, Tsang P, Leon-Garcia M, et al. Over half of the WHO guidelines published from 2014 to 2019 explicitly considered health equity issues: a cross-sectional survey. J Clin Epidemiol 2020;127:125–33.
38. Alonso-Coello P, Oxman AD, Moberg J, et al. GRADE Evidence to Decision (EtD) frameworks: a systematic and transparent approach to making well informed healthcare choices. 2: Clinical practice guidelines. BMJ 2016;353:i2089.
39. Welch VA, Akl EA, Guyatt G, et al. GRADE equity guidelines 1: considering health equity in GRADE guideline development: introduction and rationale. J Clin Epidemiol 2017;90:59–67.
40. Welch VA, Akl EA, Pottie K, et al. GRADE equity guidelines 3: considering health equity in GRADE guideline development: rating the certainty of synthesized evidence. J Clin Epidemiol 2017;90:76–83.
41. Pottie K, Welch V, Morton R, et al. GRADE equity guidelines 4: considering health equity in GRADE guideline development: evidence to decision process. J Clin Epidemiol 2017;90:84–91.
42. Barnabe C, Pianarosa E, Hazlewood G. Informing the GRADE evidence to decision process with health equity considerations: demonstration from the Canadian rheumatoid arthritis care context. J Clin Epidemiol 2021;138:147–55.
43. Pianarosa E, Hazlewood GS, Thomas M, et al. Supporting equity in rheumatoid arthritis outcomes in canada: population-specific factors in patient-centered care. J Rheumatol 2021;48:1793–802.
44. Umaefulam V, Kleissen T, Barnabe C. The representation of Indigenous peoples in chronic disease clinical trials in Australia, Canada, New Zealand, and the United States. Clin Trials 2022;19(1):22–32.
45. Woodward EN, Singh RS, Ndebele-Ngwenya P, et al. A more practical guide to incorporating health equity domains in implementation determinant frameworks. Implement Sci Commun 2021;2:61.

Printed and bound by CPI Group (UK) Ltd, Croydon, CR0 4YY

08/05/2025

01864718-0001